Death is in the Breeze:
Disease during the American Civil War

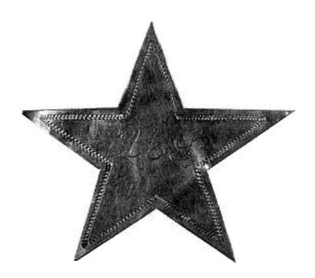

Bonnie Brice Dorwart, M.D.

2009

© Copyright 2009 by Bonnie Brice Dorwart, M.D., and the National Museum of Civil War Medicine

All rights reserved. No part of this book may be used or reproduced without written permission of the author and the publisher, except in the case of brief quotations embodied in critical essays and reviews.

Published by: The NMCWM Press
                     The National Museum of Civil War Medicine, Inc.
                     P.O. Box 470
                     Frederick, MD 21705
                     Phone: 1-800-564-1864
                     Fax: 1-301-695-6823
                     www.civilwarmed.org
                     email: museum@civilwarmed.org

ISBN-10   0-9712233-6-X
ISBN-13   978-0-9712233-6-3

The NMCWM is a not-for-profit 501(c)(3) corporation

Book design by: Scott Edie, E Graphics

Printed by: 48HrBooks.com

Printed and bound in the United States of America

First Edition

Acknowledgements

In addition to the many colleagues and patients acknowledged in the text, heartfelt thanks are due to the following:

Gary S. Daum, M.D., and Michael A. Manko, M.D., at the Lankenau Hospital, Wynnewood, PA, for providing clarification of the infectious diseases that dominated the Civil War.

Mazen Hassan, M.D., at the Walter and Leonore Annenberg Conference Center for Medical Education at Lankenau Hospital, for finding and retrieving many sources shelved long ago.

Mr. Christopher Stanwood, Ms. Lisa Gensel, Mr. Charles Greifenstein, and Mr. Richard Fraser for research assistance and document retrieval at the Historical Library of the College of Physicians of Philadelphia.

Ms. Gretchen Worden, deceased, for photographic and archival assistance in researching the holdings at the Mütter Museum of Philadelphia.

Ms. Nancy Miller and Mr. James C. Ayers, of the University of Pennsylvania Archives and Records Center in Philadelphia, for providing names and state of origin of class members, titles of graduation theses, course titles and professors in the University of Pennsylvania School of Medicine from 1849 to 1851.

Mary McGonigle, D.O.; Moira Burke, M.D.; J. Edward Pickering, M.D.; Mrs. Elizabeth Dyke, R.N.; Ms. Marie A. Norton, deceased; Ms. Gwen Clendenning; Mrs. Rose Ernst; Mrs. Anne Slater; and Mr. Norman Spielberg, for the loan of historical sources of the period.

F. Terry Hambrecht, M.D., for assistance in locating Walter Brice's commission and passage of the Medical Examining Board in Tennessee.

Peter Brodfuehrer, Ph.D., for assistance in understanding behavior of the human leech.

Nancy L. Matus, M.D., and Herbert Leavitt, M.D., deceased, for providing photographs of sexually-transmitted diseases.

Alfred Jay Bollet, M.D., Peter D'Onofrio, Ph.D., and Robert Slawson, M.D., for reviewing the manuscript.

Terry Reimer, my editor, for invaluable assistance and the staff of the NMCWM for assistance in proofreading.

H. Ralph Schumacher, Jr., M.D., for writing the Foreword.

William V. Dorwart, Jr., Ph.D., for insight into matters chemical, and for endless encouragement.

It should be noted that some of the tables and material in Chapter V were taken from two articles I wrote for the *Journal of Civil War Medicine*. The articles are: Rheumatic Diseases During the U.S. Civil War: Arthritis following Diarrhea or Dysentery. *J. Civil War Medicine* 8:13–16 (2004); and Rheumatic Diseases During the U.S. Civil War: Rheumatic Fever. *J. Civil War Medicine* 8:67–76 (2004).

This book is dedicated to my great-grandfather, Walter Brice, M.D., and to my father, Gratien Bertrand Brice, M.D., who cared for the sick and wounded soldiers of the Civil War, and of World War II.

Table of Contents

Foreword		xii
Preface		xiii
Introduction		15
Chapter I.	The Star from Shiloh	17
Chapter II.	The Making of a Civil War Surgeon	18
Chapter III.	Disease Steals through the Camps	22
Chapter IV.	Diarrhea and Dysentery: Bloody, but not from Bullets	35
Chapter V.	Rheumatism: Soldiers in Bed, not in Battle	38
Chapter VI.	Bronchitis and Catarrh	80
Chapter VII.	Abscesses, Carbuncles and Boils	83
Chapter VIII.	Mercury without Venus: Mercurials in the Treatment of Non-venereal Diseases	87
Chapter IX.	Mercury after Venus: The use of Mercury to Treat Syphilis	106
Chapter X.	How did Civil War Surgeons Keep Current with the Medical Advances of their Day?	109
Chapter XI.	Implementing and Accruing Medical Knowledge: Not a Simple Matter	112
Chapter XII.	The Legacy of Civil War Surgeons	115
Epilogue		117
Appendices		118
Bibliography		162
Index		167

Appendices

Appendix I.	Selected References on Surgery During the Civil War	118
Appendix II.	Essay Titles of 166 Students in the Class of 1851 at the University of Pennsylvania School of Medicine	119
Appendix III.	Frequency of Rheumatic Diseases During the U.S. Civil War: Tonsillitis and Heart Disease	122
Appendix IV.	Treatment of Septic Arthritis, Tracing the History of each Component, from the Text in Chapter V	127
Appendix V.	Prevention and Treatment of Gonorrhea during the Civil War	130
Appendix VI.	Preparations of Mercury Still in Use	133
Appendix VII.	Surgeries Performed with Ether or Chloroform 1847–1848 by Faculty of University of Pennsylvania School of Medicine and Jefferson Medical College	134
Appendix VIII.	History of Smallpox Prophylaxis	136
Appendix IX.	Inflammation	139
Appendix X.	Classification of Medications and Pertinent Passages from *Carson's Materia Medica of 1851*	140
Appendix XI.	Using the Broadfoot Index of 1991 to Access the Original Six-volumes of *The Medical and Surgical History of the War of the Rebellion (1861–1865)*	146
Appendix XII.	Excerpts from Lectures Heard by Walter Brice, M.D., at the University of Pennsylvania School of Medicine 1849–1851, and the Professors who gave Them	148

Illustrations

Title page
The Star from Shiloh — i

Chapter III
Figure 1. *Report of the Sick and Wounded* used by the Confederate States Army — 30

Chapter V

Figure 1.	Streptococcal sore throat	42
Figure 2.	"Smoke rings" of erythema marginatum skin rash	43
Figure 3.	Sexually acquired reactive arthritis of the thumb and ankle	52
Figure 4.	X-ray of the foot showing spur in "lover's heel"	53
Figure 5.	Mild balanitis in a patient with reactive arthritis	53
Figure 6.	Severe balanitis in reactive arthritis	53
Figure 7.	Mild conjunctivitis of both eyes in reactive arthritis	54
Figure 8.	Severe conjunctivitis of right eye in reactive arthritis	54
Figure 9.	Natural history of deformities in ankylosing spondylitis	55
Figure 10.	World War II veteran with ankylosing spondylitis	56
Figure 11.	Tuberculosis of the thoracic spine, post-mortem specimen	58
Figure 12.	Tuberculosis of the right sterno-clavicular joint	59
Figure 13.	Lymph nodes infected with tuberculosis in a Viet Nam veteran	59
Figure 14.	Tuberculosis of the right elbow joint	59
Figure 15.	Septic arthritis of the right elbow of a Viet Nam veteran	61
Figure 16.	Staphylococci in pus from right elbow as seen under the microscope	62
Figure 17.	Typical urethral discharge of gonorrhea	63
Figure 18.	Gonococcal arthritis of the left knee	63
Figure 19.	Fingertip "blood blister" of gonococcal arthritis acquired by men having sex with men	64
Figure 20.	The chancre (ulcer) of primary syphilis	65
Figure 21.	The "mucous patches" on the tongue of secondary syphilis	66
Figure 22.	Syringe of the Civil War period	68
Figure 23.	Rheumatoid arthritis involving both knees in a Viet Nam veteran	69
Figure 24.	Longstanding deformities of rheumatoid arthritis in a Korean War veteran	69
Figure 25.	The female anopheles mosquito, vector of malaria	70

| Figure 26. | Gout involving multiple joints in a Korean War veteran | 72 |

Chapter VIII

Figure 1.	Rectum of Civil War soldier who died of dysentery	88
Figure 2.	Pneumonia, gross pathological specimen	91
Figure 3.	The human leech, used to remove blood believed to contain substances that caused sickness in soldiers of the Civil War	92
Figure 4.	Mercury thermometer of the Civil War period	96
Figure 5.	Self-registering thermometer, invented in 1870	96
Figure 6.	Colon of a Civil War soldier with dysentery, treated twice with mercury	101
Figure 7.	Colon from another soldier with dysentery not prescribed mercury	101

Appendix XII

Figure 1.	Nathaniel Chapman, M.D. (1780–1853)	150
Figure 2.	William E. Horner, M.D. (1793–1853)	150
Figure 3.	George B. Wood, M.D. (1797–1879)	150
Figure 4.	James B. Rogers, M.D. (1802–1852)	150
Figure 5.	William Gibson, M.D. (1788–1868)	150
Figure 6.	Hugh L. Hodge, M.D. (1796–1873)	150
Figure 7.	Samuel Jackson, M.D. (1787–1872)	150
Figure 8.	Joseph Carson, M.D. (1808–1876)	150

Tables

Chapter III

Table I.	Leading Causes of Sickness, July 1, 1861–June 30, 1862, U.S. Army, White Troops	26
Table II.	Causes of Sickness, July 1, 1862–June 30, 1863, U.S. Army, White Troops	26
Table III.	Causes of Sickness, July 1, 1863–June 30, 1864, U.S. Army, White Troops	26
Table IV.	Causes of Sickness, July 1, 1864–June 30, 1865, U.S. Army, White Troops	27
Table V.	Causes of Sickness, First Year after the War, July 1, 1865–June 30, 1866, U.S. Army, White Troops	27
Table VI.	Causes of Sickness in U.S. Colored Troops, July 1, 1863–June 30, 1864, in Atlantic and Central Regions	27
Table VII.	Causes of Sickness, July 1, 1864–June 30, 1865, All Regions, U.S. Colored Troops	28
Table VIII.	Causes of Sickness, July 1, 1865–June 30, 1866, All Regions, U.S. Colored Troops	28
Table IX.	Leading Causes of Sickness and Resulting Deaths, July 1, 1861–June 30, 1866, U.S. Army White Troops	29
Table X.	Leading Causes of Sickness and Resulting Deaths, July 1, 1863–June 30, 1866, U.S. Colored Troops	29
Table XI.	Cases of Sickness and Wounds from Certain of the CSA during Portions of the Years 1861, 1862 and 1863, with the Corresponding Rates of the Army of the Potomac (USA) for nine months ending March 1862	32

Chapter IV

Table I.	Cases of Diarrhea/Dysentery per 1,000 Mean Troop Strength, all years	35

Chapter V

Table I.	Cases of Rheumatism per 1,000 Mean Troop Strength, all years	39
Table II.	Jones Criteria for Diagnosis of Rheumatic Fever, 1944	41
Table III.	Diagnostic Criteria for Rheumatic Fever, 1992	41
Table IV.	Arthritis Attributed to Gout	71
Table V.	Outcome of 44 Cases of Rheumatism Reported by the Union Army	73

Table VI.	Outcome of Cases of Rheumatism Listed in the *Sickness and Mortality Reports*	73
Table VII.	Mortality from Rheumatism in General Hospitals, Union Army in Two Regions	73
Table VIII.	Discharge on Surgeon's Certificate of Disability of those with Rheumatic Diseases	74
Table IX.	Reasons for Discharge with Disability in U.S. White Troops, Total for the War	74
Table X.	Reasons for Discharge with Disability in U.S. Colored Troops, Total for the War	74

Chapter VI

Table I.	Frequency of the Common Cold by Month the First Year of the War	81
Table II.	Frequency of Colds/Acute Bronchitis by Month the Second Year of the War	82

Chapter VII

Table I.	Cases of Abscesses, Carbuncles or Boils in all Years of the War	83

Chapter VIII

Table I.	Outcomes of Treatment with Mercury	93

Appendices

Table I.	Tonsillitis. Army of the United States, Year ending 6–30–1862	122
Table II.	Tonsillitis. Army of the United States, 7–1–1862 to 6–30–1863	122
Table III.	Tonsillitis. Army of the United States, 7–1–1863 to 6–30–1864	122
Table IV.	Tonsillitis. Army of the United States, 7–1–1864 to 6–30–1865	123
Table V.	Tonsillitis. Army of the United States, 7–1–1865 to 6–30–1866	123
Table VI.	Tonsillitis. Army of the United States, (Colored Troops), 7–1–1863 to 6–30–1864	123
Table VII.	Tonsillitis. Army of the United States, (Colored Troops), 7–1–1864 to 6–30–1865	123
Table VIII.	Tonsillitis. Army of the United States, (Colored Troops), 7–1–1865 to 6–30–1866	124
Table IX.	Heart disease. Army of the United States, Year Ending 6–30–1862	124

Table X.	Heart disease. Army of the United States, 7–1–1862 to 6–30–1863	124
Table XI.	Heart disease. Army of the United States, 7–1–1863 to 6–30–1864	124
Table XII.	Heart disease. Army of the United States, 7–1–1864 to 6–30–1865	125
Table XIII.	Heart disease. Army of the United States, 7–1–1865 to 6–30–1866	125
Table XIV.	Heart disease. Army of the United States, (Colored Troops) 7–1–1863 to 6–30–1864	125
Table XV.	Heart disease. Army of the United States, (Colored Troops) 7–1–1864 to 6–30–1865	125
Table XVI.	Heart disease. Army of the United States, (Colored Troops) 7–1–1865 to 6–30–1866	126

Foreword

Both the American Civil War and medical history have fascinated many. This tour de force, by Dr. Bonnie Dorwart, combines these two areas in a unique analysis of medicine during the United States Civil War. This important addition to writings about Civil War medicine provides descriptions of lectures the military surgeons received in medical school. Dr. Dorwart points out that even the most prestigious schools provided mostly opinions based on experience with a frequent emphasis on the role of "bad air" in the pathogenesis of many diseases. This was the state of the art but left the young doctors ill prepared by any of our current concepts for what they were to deal with on the battlefields and in the camps. This background makes some of the success stories even more dramatic. Deaths were due to the wounds of battle but much more often due to disease related in large part to crowded camps with little attention to sanitation.

Dr. Dorwart's interest has obviously been stimulated by the fact that her great-grandfather was a Confederate surgeon in the war. His and his colleagues' stories, backgrounds, and later accomplishments culled from original sources make for fascinating reading.

As a fellow rheumatologist, I am intrigued by Dr. Dorwart's observations on the importance of rheumatic fever during the war. She has also dredged up descriptions of arthritis following dysentery and urethritis that suggest reactive arthritis long before the first accepted descriptions during World War I.

As you read this, you will be both appalled by the horrors and enthralled by the efforts made by physicians on both sides. Many therapies such as purging and mercury may have hastened deaths. What will our successors think of our efforts 150 years from now?

H. Ralph Schumacher, Jr., M.D.
Professor of Medicine, University of Pennsylvania

Preface

The title of this work was inspired by a speaker on behalf of the United States Sanitary Commission, who exhorted the citizenry of New York: "We beg you to awake to instant action. Disease, insidious and inevitable, is now stealing through the camps, on scorching plain, in midnight damp, menacing our dearest treasure—the very flower of the nation's youth. Death is already in the breeze."[1]

The star on the title page is a photograph of an insignia removed from a Union soldier who died at Shiloh. Passed down in my family, it cried out for several questions to be answered: Who was that soldier? Could his family be found and the star returned to them?

The recipient of the star was my great-grandfather, Walter Brice, M.D. His history—before and after Shiloh—offers an insight into the medical education and experiences of the Civil War surgeon. Walter Brice was mustered in at Jackson, Tennessee, as Assistant Surgeon in the Tennessee 9th Infantry Regiment of the Confederate States Army (CSA). After the battle of Shiloh, he was elected as Regimental Surgeon of the Tennessee 9th Infantry, and later of the Tennessee 6th Infantry Regiment. He received an M.D. degree from the University of Pennsylvania School of Medicine in Philadelphia in 1851, as did his classmate, the noted Union surgeon, George A. Otis, Jr. Graduating from that institution three years before Brice, Samuel H. Stout served as Medical Director of Hospitals for the Confederate Army of Tennessee. In 1853 Joseph J. Woodward, the extraordinary Union Army surgeon who wrote much of the *Medical and Surgical History of the War of the Rebellion* (1861–1865), received an M.D. degree from the same school.

The Jefferson Medical College, also in Philadelphia, awarded the M.D. at nearly the same time to other Union Army greats Jonathan Letterman (1849), S. Weir Mitchell (1850) and George R. Morehouse (1850). The lectures that Walter Brice heard survive today and detail what physicians caring for soldiers in the U.S. Civil War were taught. These archives also record how medical students were trained scientifically and ethically to enter medicine as a calling and as a profession. Dr. Walter Brice achieved no great distinction, but others who studied medicine contemporaneously, some of whom are listed above, did. Lectures delivered three years before and two years after those to Brice did not vary. His medical education was their medical education. Indeed, one of his influential professors, Joseph Carson, published four essentially identical editions of his text on pharmacology between 1851 and 1867.

By the time Brice entered medical school, he had attended the Field School in Fairfield County, South Carolina. At 13 years of age "he was sufficiently advanced in Latin, Greek and the sciences to enter the freshman class of Erskine College at Due West, South Carolina." He graduated at 18 with honors.[2] Required to study with a physician before applying to medical school, he studied with his uncle, also named Walter Brice, from 1848 to 1849. His uncle graduated from Jefferson College, Canonsburg, Pennsylvania, in 1828 and from the Medical College [now the Medical University] of South Carolina, Charleston, in 1831.

The premedical education of both was unusual for that time, the requirements for admission to medical school being far less stringent than those they imposed on themselves. Indeed, as late as 1910, the University of Pennsylvania School of Medicine required only "one year of college work, in which, however, conditions have been very freely allowed."[3] At

xiii

the same time Jefferson Medical College required for entrance "a high school education or its equivalent."[4] In Chapter II we shall examine in more detail the education of a surgeon of the Civil War.

Preface References

1. *Documents of the U.S. Sanitary Commission #16*, Vol. I, New York: U.S. Sanitary Commission; 1866: 1–2
2. Brice JM. Tribute to Dr. Walter Brice on the event of his Death. Union City, TN: *The News Banner*; November 9, 1895
3. Flexner A. *Medical Education in the United States and Canada*. Boston: D.B. Updike, Merrymount Press; 1910: 293
4. *Ibid.*, 294

Introduction

This book is intended for a general audience, for the curious reader who is familiar with the various campaigns and battles fought during the Civil War, but who is not necessarily a physician, and would like to learn more about the diseases that killed twice as many soldiers as weapons did. In the past half-century several superb books have been written about medicine as it was practiced during the war. Examples are George W. Adams' *Doctors in Blue* (1952), Howard H. Cunningham's *Doctors in Gray* (1958), Paul E. Steiner's, *Disease in the Civil War* (1968), Frank R. Freemon's *Microbes and Minié Balls* (1993), Robert E. Denney's *Civil War Medicine: Care & Comfort of the Wounded* (1995), Alfred Jay Bollet's *Civil War Medicine: Challenges and Triumphs* (2002), Michael A. Flannery's *Civil War Pharmacy: A History of Drugs, Drug Supply and Provision, and Therapeutics for the Union and Confederacy* (2004) and Ira M. Rutkow's *Bleeding Blue and Gray: Civil War Surgery and the Evolution of American Medicine* (2005).

Readers who wish to learn about surgery during the War will find little in the present book, since it focuses on medical conditions caused by disease. Surgery of the time dealt, of course, with the wounds suffered by soldiers. Surgeons cleared foreign bodies from wounds, tied off bleeding arteries and veins, amputated limbs or portions thereof when decay of the destroyed tissue assured fatal infections, and drained abscesses. What they did not do was electively repair simple hernias or perform appendectomies, because entry into the abdominal cavity ensured almost certain death from infection. They could not operate in the chest either, since breathing could not be supported and infection was a near certainty there as well.

An excellent introduction to the surgical skills demanded during and after battle can be found in Dr. Clyde B. Kernek's 1993 book, *Field Surgeon at Gettysburg*. His book also provides an insight into the operation of the superb ambulance system devised by Dr. Jonathan Letterman—under command of the Medical, not the Quartermaster, Department. Dr. Kernek also walks the reader through staged care on the battlefield—initially at a field station, then a field hospital and finally a general hospital, when appropriate for care of the soldier. Also for the reader interested in surgery during the War, there are several period works that can still be found today in comprehensive historical collections such as those at the College of Physicians of Philadelphia. These include:

Manual of Surgery, by Astley Cooper and Joseph Henry Green, ed. Thomas Castle (Charles S. Francis, New York, 1839)

Illustrated manual of operative surgery and surgical anatomy, a volume of 513 pages and 88 colored plates, by Claude Bernard and Charles Hutted (Publisher Billiard Brothers, New York, 1861)

A practical treatise on military surgery, by Frank Hastings Hamilton (Billiard Brothers, New York, 1861)

Hand-book of surgical operations, by Stephen Smith (Billiard Brothers, New York, 1862)

The three massive surgical volumes of *The Medical and Surgical History of the War of the Rebellion*, published by The U.S. Government Printing Office in 1875, 1877 and 1883, containing thousands of illustrations of wounds and surgical specimens, and descriptions of surgical procedures.

A manual of military surgery, for the use of surgeons in the Confederate Army, by J. Julian Chisholm (Evans & Cogswell, Charleston S.C., 1861).

It is interesting to note that in this last work on military surgery, Dr. Chisholm's 1864 edition (page 121) nonetheless emphasizes the importance of medical entities: The "fire of an enemy never decimates an opposing army. Disease is the fell destroyer of armies, and stalks at all times through encampments. Where balls have destroyed hundreds, insidious diseases, with their long train of symptoms, and quiet, noiseless progress, sweep away thousands. To keep an army in health is, then, even more important than to cure wounds from the battlefields." Appendix I of my book lists other publications that detail surgical instruments, procedures performed, braces, and prosthetic devices for amputees in the Civil War.

The present work, a product of six years of research using primary sources of the 1840s, 1850s, and 1860s, focuses on the pharmacopoeias, medical dictionaries, textbooks, scientific journals, and lectures available to doctors and medical students of the time—what physicians caring for soldiers in the war knew, and when they knew it. The book also looks at how medical conditions encountered by the Civil War surgeon were treated then, how those entities would be treated now, and when knowledge leading to current therapies became available.

A major cause of the inability of soldiers to fight, rheumatism, has not been written about in detail. As a rheumatologist, I feel this is a subject worthy of study and have devoted much of the text to it.

Mercury is touted as a major part of the therapeutic arsenal of the Civil War surgeon, yet I was unable to find a systematic analysis of conditions in which it was prescribed and how often it was used. Therefore, there is a sizeable section devoted to this subject. To permit the physicians of that time to speak for themselves, original case reports and commentary are frequently and liberally quoted instead of being paraphrased.

Chapter I.
The Star from Shiloh

A shiny brass star was part of my family's history, along with genealogical charts, obituaries, gravestone inscriptions, family crests and a microscope. What was not known was who wore the star at the Battle of Shiloh during the U.S. Civil War. The hunt for its owner began in earnest in 1998, with research into the military history of Walter Brice, my great-grandfather, whose initial service was at Shiloh. The star, according to my ancestors, was removed from a Union general who died during the battle and given to Brice. Appalled that the star was taken as a war souvenir, Assistant Surgeon Brice returned to the battlefield to replace it on the General's uniform. Unfortunately the body had been moved.

Initially the story sounded plausible. Only one Union General, William H.L. Wallace, died at Shiloh, and he was a one-star (Brigadier) General. He was wounded at Sunken Road on April 6, 1862.[1] Taken for dead by his own troops, his body was moved to safety during the battle; he was found the next day, alive. General Wallace died on April 10.[2] I knew, however, that the rank of Union and Confederate officers was indicated, not by metallic insignias, but by cloth ones sewn on their uniforms. Puzzled, I contacted Stacy Allen, historian at the Shiloh National Military Park. He informed me that my star was technically called a brass ray, which most likely belonged to a Texas soldier, and was worn on the hat, not on the shoulder. It did not match any in the Park's collection.[3] This explanation appears reasonable. The lone star had been a symbol of Texas since its placement on the 1836 flag of the Republic of Texas, and the uniforms of many soldiers in early battles like Shiloh were not yet standardized. A Texas private could well have been mistaken for a Union general. The *US* engraving on the star indicates it was of pre-war issue.

Having "struck out" pursuing the brass ray, but fascinated by what little I had already learned, I turned my attention to the family member who was given the star. That person was Walter Brice, M.D., who, living in western Tennessee, volunteered to be a soldier in the Confederate Army. This book is the outgrowth of my research on him.

Chapter I References

1. Daniel, L.J. *Shiloh: The Battle That Changed the Civil War*. New York: Simon & Schuster; 1997:232
2. *Ibid.*, 231
3. Allen S. Personal communication: February 4, 1999

Chapter II.

The Making of a Civil War Surgeon

In Walter Brice's class at the University of Pennsylvania School of Medicine in 1851, 58% of the student body of 167 came from southern states, as follows: Tennessee (10 students), Virginia (25), Mississippi (10), North Carolina (22), South Carolina (1), Georgia (2), Kentucky (8), Alabama (5), Louisiana (7), Maryland (6), and Florida (1).[1]

There were nine medical schools in the southern United States that Walter Brice and his classmates from the South could have attended in 1849. These include Medical College of South Carolina, Charleston; Medical College of Georgia, Augusta; University of Virginia, Department of Medicine, Charlottesville; Medical College of Virginia, Richmond; Medical Department of the Tulane University of Louisiana, New Orleans; University of Louisville Medical Department, Louisville; University of Maryland School of Medicine, Baltimore; George Washington University, Department of Medicine, District of Columbia; and Washington University Medical Department, St. Louis.[2]

Instead, they chose to come to the University of Pennsylvania School of Medicine in Philadelphia, established exactly a century before the Civil War ended. It is likely, although not certain, that all returned to practice medicine in the South. That such a large number came North to study ensured uniformity in the medical training of many of the doctors soon to be caring for soldiers on both sides of the armed conflict.

The medical school of the University of Pennsylvania is the oldest such institution in the United States. Initially it was called the Medical School of the College of Philadelphia when founded by John Morgan in 1765. Later, the school became the School of Medicine of the University of Pennsylvania, which had been established in 1735.[3] "Rules" of the University of Pennsylvania required Walter Brice, age 19, to attend lectures in the fall and spring for two years.[4] Subjects for the 1849–1850 session were *Theory and Practice of Medicine, Anatomy, Materia Medica and Pharmacy, Chemistry, Surgery, Obstetrics and the Diseases of Women and Children*, and *Institutes of Medicine*.

Because of a custom of the time, viewed as peculiar and quaint now, the very lectures that Walter Brice heard were published. If medical students deemed a lecture important, they collected money from the class and paid to have the lecture published. From these one gleans considerable information about medical education during the pre-Civil War period, at least in Philadelphia. Students were taught that science is based on judging the correct answer to a problem and on experience. Experimentation in a laboratory is not mentioned. There is no notion of controlled trials, even though English naval physician, James Lind, published one in 1753 in *A Treatise on the Scurvy*, and no concept of evidence-based medicine. Neither were the students told about another physician, Pierre C.A. Louis, who published a study only fifteen years before, comparing the outcomes of consecutive patients with pneumonia treated by bleeding with those who were not. He showed that there was no difference in survival.

Furthermore, these students were still taught that a "life force" was needed to direct the functions of the body,[5] despite the findings of Friedrich Wöhler in 1828 that no such force was required. Wöhler accomplished the synthesis of urea, which previously had been made only by living things, from ammonium cyanate, an inorganic compound.[6] Evidently it took some time for the world of medicine to catch up to that of chemistry. One reason why Wöhler's seminal contributions might not have reached Philadelphia was that the 1828 paper was published in German, and his textbook on organic chemistry in French, Dutch, Danish, and Swedish, but not in English.[7] In fact, the idea of the life force (called *vitalism*), that only living things could create organic compounds, would not be debunked finally until 1865, when Claude Bernard showed that physical and chemical reactions alone permitted all the body's functions to occur and did not require any mysterious invisible vital force to do so.

Walter Brice and classmates learned during their second and final year in medical school the role of hygiene and crowding in causing disease, but these are couched in terms of "bad air" produced by humans or arising from the earth.[8] This inability to conceive of *particles* as causes of infections would hamper the ability of Civil War surgeons (all doctors were called surgeons during the war) to prevent the most common and deadly diseases among their patients. After all, one can control particles—by washing them off surfaces or clothing, brushing them away, killing them with toxic chemicals, isolating human carriers who harbor them, eliminating their vectors with screens or nets, burying dead matter, or draining still water on which they might feed or breed. But what can one do to control air? The spectacular insights and experiments that indicted particles as the cause of infection—living particles, no less—by Pasteur (1861–1880), Lister (1867) and Koch (1877) occurred after the war. The role of causative agents, vectors, intermediate hosts, and carriers—people who, despite showing no signs of illness, can transmit disease—were all unknown until the last two decades of the nineteenth century and the early part of the twentieth century.

Walter Brice's professors instilled in their students destined to become Civil War surgeons the ethics of medicine, a desire to care for their fellow man, and the necessity of continuing medical education throughout life. They taught them with dedication and preparation the science of the day.[9] Medical students educated in the South received similar instruction. Joseph Jones, M.D., was a distinguished Confederate surgeon and an influential medical author and historian of the war. In 1859 he was Professor of Medical Chemistry and Pharmacy at the Medical College of Georgia in Augusta. At least one of his lectures survives because his students judged it worthy of publication. Jones emphasized chemistry, math, physics and the inter-relationships of medicine to these other sciences.[10]

Several medical schools of the day required students to write a senior thesis in order to graduate. Titles of those from the Class of 1851 of the University of Pennsylvania School of Medicine, shown in Appendix II, provide another unique window into the training of physicians in the mid-nineteenth century. A decade later they would find their skills ill suited to serving in the military in the war which claimed more lives than any other, before or since, in United States history. In fact, their woefully inadequate medical training reflected the fact that in the 100 years before the Civil War there were only three significant medical advances—vaccination against smallpox, anesthesia with chloroform and ether, and the discovery by Oliver Wendell Holmes, Sr., and Ignaz Philipp Semmelweis that fatal infections were caused by doctors who failed to wash their hands between examinations of patients. Anesthesia and, to an extent, smallpox prevention, were used during the war; alas the importance of hand washing—published in a German journal in 1847—was virtually unknown to them.

Chapter II

Prior to the secession of South Carolina from the United States on December 20, 1860, there was a small Regular Army. It consisted of 1,117 commissioned officers and 11,907 enlisted men. Union Surgeon D. L. Huntington described its Medical Department thus:

> The Medical Department was composed of one Surgeon General with the rank of Colonel; thirty Surgeons with the rank of Major, and eighty-four Assistant Surgeons holding for the first five years the rank of 1st Lieutenant, and subsequent to that period, until promotion to Surgeon, the rank of Captain. The officers of the Medical Department formed a portion of the General Staff of the army; were not permanently attached to any regiment or command, but were subject to duty wherever their services were needed. Experience had demonstrated this system to be the best for the necessities of an army widely scattered over an immense area of territory, serving in commands of less than regimental strength [1,000 men in a regiment].[11]

After Lincoln called for help in controlling the rebellion in 1861, large numbers of State troops, or militia, were raised:

> Each regiment was provided with a Surgeon and an Assistant Surgeon commissioned by the States in which the troops had been enlisted. These officers were borne on the muster-rolls and permanently attached to the regimental organization, being seldom detached except for urgent reasons.[11]

By the end of the war 547 Surgeons and Assistant Surgeons of Volunteers were appointed. Mustered into service were 2,109 regimental Surgeons and 3,882 regimental Assistant Surgeons. In addition were employed 85 Acting Staff Surgeons and 5,532 Acting Assistant Surgeons,[12] who served as "contract surgeons" in the general hospitals.

A monumental change in the structure of the Medical Department of the Union Army was effected in an act of Congress on April 16, 1862, wherein the rank of the Surgeon General was raised from Colonel to that of Brigadier General, giving him rank that assured control by the Medical Department of all aspects of patient care and welfare in the Union Army. Section 4 of that same act rid the army of disorganized senescent high-ranking medical officers who achieved their rank by seniority and not by ability. It provided:

> That the Surgeon General, the Assistant Surgeon General, Medical Inspector General, and medical inspectors, shall, immediately…be appointed by the President, by and with the advice and consent of the Senate, by selection from the medical corps of the army, or from the surgeons in the volunteer service, *without regard to their rank…, but with sole regard to qualifications.* [Emphasis added][13]

Nine days later Lincoln appointed William A. Hammond, M.D., Surgeon General, replacing Acting Surgeon General Robert Wood.

The South was most fortunate in having a single competent, albeit brusque, Surgeon General, Samuel Preston Moore, from July 30, 1861, until the conclusion of the war. A member of the Medical Department of the United States Army prior to the war, Moore, not surprisingly, structured the Medical Department of the Confederate Army in much the same way.[14] The:

> Total number of medical officers in the Confederate Army has been estimated at 834 Surgeons and 1,668 Assistant Surgeons; there were an estimated seventy-three medical officers in the Confederate Navy. Unlike the Union Medical Department initially bogged down with old hangers-on, the Confederate medical corps had no traditions placing its officers in an administrative straitjacket.[15]

In the next chapter, the prologue ends, and the War begins.

Chapter II References

1. Horner WE. *Medical Commencement of the University of Pennsylvania held on Saturday, April 5, 1851: with a Valedictory by W. E. Horner, M.D., Professor of Anatomy.* Philadelphia: L.R. Bailey, Printer; 1851: 3–8

2. Slawson RG. *Medical Training in the United States Prior to the Civil War.* Tenth Annual Conference on Civil War Medicine, Shepherdstown, WV, Aug. 2–4, 2002

3. Bayne-Jones S. *The evolution of preventive medicine in the U.S. Army, 1607–1939.* Washington: US Government Printing Office; 1968: 23

4. *Catalogue of the Trustees, Officers & Students of the University of Pennsylvania, Session 1850–51.* Philadelphia: L.R. Bailey, Printer; 1851: 36

5. Jackson S. *An introductory lecture, preliminary to a course on the Institutes of Medicine, delivered on the 9th of October, 1850, before the class of the University of Pennsylvania.* Philadelphia: Journeymen Printers' Office; 1850: 14

6. Wöhler F. *Annalen der Physik und Chemie,* 2nd series 12; 1828: 252–256

7. Friedrich Wohler, in *Dictionary of Scientific Biography*, ed. Gillispie CC. Charles Scribner's Sons, NY; 1981. 13: 475, 478

8. Jackson S. *An introductory lecture, preliminary to a course on the University of Pennsylvania.* Philadelphia: Journeymen Printers' Office; 1850: 16

9. Horner WE. *Medical Commencement of the University of Pennsylvania held on Saturday, April 5, 1851: with a Valedictory by W. E. Horner, M.D., Professor of Anatomy.* Philadelphia: L.R. Bailey, Printer; 1851: 10

10. Jones J. *Suggestions on Medical Education. Introductory Lecture to the course of 1859–60 in the Medical College of Georgia.* Augusta, GA: Constitutionalist Book and Job Office; 1860: 5

11. *Medical and Surgical History of the Civil War.* Wilmington, NC: Broadfoot Publishing; 1990: Vol. XII 899. Hereafter *MSHCW*

12. *Ibid.*, 901

13. *Ibid.*, 900

14. Moore SP. Regulations of the Confederate States of America Medical Department, in *Regulations for the Army of the Confederate States.* Richmond: Randolph; 1862. Repub.: San Francisco: Norman Publishing, 1992: 236–258

15. Flannery MA. *Civil War Pharmacy: A History of Drugs, Drug Supply and Provision, and Therapeutics for the Union and Confederacy.* Binghamton, NY: Haworth Press, Inc.; 2004:21

Chapter III.
Disease Steals through the Camps

"Disease, insidious and inevitable, is now stealing through the camps...menacing our dearest treasure—the...nation's youth."[1]

There are four characteristics of every army which influence public health in wartime: enlisted men are males 20 to 30 years old; they live in crowded circumstances; environmental conditions in the field are primitive; and military objectives sometimes override sanitary ones.[2]

The armies who fought in the United States Civil War were comprised largely of Caucasian males who grew up in relative isolation on farms. Not having experienced the common diseases of childhood, the new soldiers fell prey to them as adults. General Lee wrote his wife, Mary Custis Lee, on August 4, 1861, "The soldiers everywhere are sick. The measles are prevalent throughout the whole army...."[3] By September 1, in another letter to Mrs. Lee, his battle readiness is still hobbled by infectious diseases affecting his troops. The General's writing underscores the severity of measles in the adult:

> We have a great deal of sickness among the soldiers, and now those on the sick-list would form an army. The measles is still among them, though I hope it is dying out. But it is a disease which though light in childhood is severe in manhood, and prepares the system for other attacks.[4]

Lee was correct in observing that measles is a serious disease in the adult. In a 1991 report to the Centers for Disease Control, complications from measles were more common in patients older than 20 years than in children.[5] In one series of 3,220 military recruits who contracted measles between 1976 and 1979, 3% developed pneumonia, requiring hospitalization. Seventeen percent had bronchitis, 31% hepatitis, 29% middle ear infection, and 25% sinusitis.[5] Many who live in the 21st century and are fortunate to have been vaccinated against measles do not realize that death can occur in the unprotected non-immunized human. Frequently pneumonia was the fatal complication of young soldiers in the Civil War who contracted measles. Eighteen-year-old Private Munck lived, but suffered deafness in one ear following his bout of measles:

> **Case 26**. —Private James A. Munck, Co. G, 100th Pa; age 18; Enlisted Feb. 5, 1864. He contracted measles and was admitted, March 27, to Division No. 1 hospital, whence he was transferred to Mower hospital, Philadelphia, and on May 13 to this hospital [Satterlee]. Diagnosis: Deafness of the right ear. Warm water was used by syringe and a few drops of a weak solution of sulphate of zinc were instilled daily into the ear. Improvement followed and the patient was returned to duty August 6. —Satterlee Hospital, Philadelphia, Pa.[6]

Mumps also is usually a more severe infection in adults than in children.

If the common contagious diseases of childhood did not strike down soldiers, diseases spread by the "four Fs"—flies, fingers, feces, and food—did. These are the illnesses caused by bacteria that maximize their reproduction when humans and unsanitary conditions coexist. Diarrhea, dysentery, typhoid fever, and food poisoning with bacteria such as *Salmonella* are direct consequences of unsanitary practices.

Environmental conditions in the field were primitive. Sometimes military objectives necessarily overrode sanitary ones. It was not because the relationship between sanitation and disease was unknown at the time of the Civil War that lapses of sanitation occurred. The sanitary reform movement preceded the war, evolving between 1800 and 1860, with publication of such works as the Shattuck report of 1850.[7]

One surgeon, Jonathan Letterman, Medical Director of the Army of the Potomac for eighteen months, was very aware of the importance of enforcing sanitation. In his *Medical Recollections of the Army of the Potomac*, he wrote:

> The duties of Medical officers are not confined to prescribing drugs, but that it is also their duty…to preserve the health of those who are well. My efforts to reduce the amount of disease to the lowest possible ratio were unceasing, and my attention was constantly given to the location and police of the camps, to the proper arrangement of the hospitals, and to the care bestowed upon the sick and wounded.[8]

Letterman addressed the problems that surgeons experienced from non-medical officers in carrying out sanitary measures:

> I am convinced that there exists in the minds of many, perhaps the majority, of line officers, a very imperfect conception of the position of Medical officers, and the objects for which a Medical Staff was instituted. It is a popular delusion that the highest duties of Medical officers are performed in prescribing a drug or amputating a limb; and the troops frequently…are compelled to endure suffering which would have been avoided did commanders take a comprehensive view of this important subject.[9]

Letterman never lost sight of the role of the surgeon—to provide his commanders with healthy soldiers who can win the war:

> A corps of Medical officers was not established solely for the purpose of attending the wounded and sick…. The leading idea…is to strengthen the hands of the commanding General by keeping his army in the most vigorous health, thus rendering it, in the highest degree, efficient for *enduring fatigue and privation, and for fighting* [emphasis added].[10]

Evidence that unsanitary conditions were common during the war. There are frequent references to the interplay of flies, fingers, feces, and food during the war.

Chapter III

Dr. Joseph Jones, the Confederate surgeon inspecting the Andersonville stockade in Sumter County, Georgia, wrote of a stream there:

> As these waters, loaded with filth and human excrement, flow sluggishly through the swamp below, filled with trees and reeds coated with a filthy deposit, they emit an intolerable and most sickening stench. Standing as I did over these waters in the middle of a hot day in September, as they rolled sluggishly forth from the stockade, after having received the filth and excrement of twenty thousand men, the stench was disgusting and overpowering; and if it was surpassed in unpleasantness by anything, it was only in the disgusting appearance of the filthy, almost stagnant, waters moving slowly between the stumps and roots and fallen trunks of trees and thick branches of reeds, with innumerable long-tailed, large white maggots, swollen peas, and fermenting excrement, and fragments of bread and meat.[11]

Equally unsanitary conditions prevailed in the Andersonville prison hospital. "Sick men, unable to visit the latrines, made use of small wooden boxes in the lanes behind the tents." Jones gave these further details:

> Millions of flies swarmed over everything and covered the faces of the sleeping patients, and crawled down their open mouths, and deposited their maggots in the gangrenous wounds of the living and in the mouths of the dead. Myriads of mosquitoes also infested the tents, and many of the patients were so stung by these pestiferous insects that they appeared as if they were suffering from a slight attack of measles.
>
> The cooking arrangements were of the most miserable and defective character. Two large iron pots similar to those used for boiling sugar-cane were the only cooking utensils furnished by the hospital for the cooking of near [sic] two thousand men; and the patients were dependent in great measure upon their own miserable utensils. They were allowed to cook in the tent-doors and in the lanes, and this was another source of filth and another favorable condition for the generation of flies and other vermin.[12]

Thomas A. McParlin, Surgeon, U.S. Army, who succeeded Jonathan Letterman as Medical Director of the Army of the Potomac, wrote about soldiers hospitalized after the battles around Cool Arbor [Cold Harbor], Virginia, in May of 1864:

> The inmates of the hospitals experienced great annoyance from dust, and from the swarms of flies which seemed to spring up everywhere. For the first evil, there could be but little remedy. A large number of musquito [sic] bars [nets] procured and distributed served to abate the latter nuisance to a great degree.[13]

Joseph J. Woodward, Surgeon, U.S. Army, documented that these same breaches of sanitation occurred in camps:

> In great armies in time of war personal cleanliness is often far from all that could be desired. How often, are the men unwashed, their clothes filthy, their bodies full of vermin, and heaps of garbage about the camp…! Especially [needed] was…policing the latrines. [The] trench is generally too shallow [not the requisite five feet deep] the daily covering…with dirt is entirely neglected. Large numbers of the men will not use the sinks [latrines], …but instead every clump of bushes, every fence border in the vicinity….It is impossible to take a step outside of the limits of the encampment… without having both eye and nostril continually offended.[14]

Assistant Surgeon H. E. Brown, U.S. Army, after the Battle of Seven Pines (Fair Oaks), Virginia, May 31–June 1, 1862, reported on camp conditions, "Over 3000 dead had been buried…. Dead horses, insufficiently buried or burnt, filled the air with a noxious effluvium, and the only water was infiltrated with the decaying animal matter of the battlefield."[15]

Dr. Newberry, in a United States Sanitary Commission (U.S.S.C.) report from the Mississippi Valley in late 1861, documented contamination of the water supply with the soldiers' excrement. "The sink [latrine] is the ground in the vicinity, which slopes down to the stream, from which all water in the camp is obtained."[16] Dr. Aigner amplified further on camp conditions in Cairo, Illinois, in the same report. "The horses and mules are invariably kept too near the camps, and the daily removal of their dung is a myth dreamed of only by the authors of the army regulations and the Sanitary Commission Inspectors."[17] Estimating that a horse produces 30 pounds of feces daily, and that an army of 50,000 men might be accompanied by 15,000 horses and mules, one can imagine the enormous task posed by covering or burying the daily dung.

For those spared childhood infections or diseases associated with poor hygiene, malaria could be counted on to cause dangerous fevers and liver disease whenever stagnant water abounded.

The role played by malaria. The cause of malaria—a parasite—and its mode of transmission by the anopheles mosquito was not determined until 1897, three decades after the Civil War ended. Numerous accounts attest to the presence of the vector, although it was recognized only as a nuisance at that time. From the *U.S.S.C. Report #69* of 1863, it is clear that mosquitoes were such an aggravation to the troops immediately after the Battle of Gettysburg that the great expenditure of $810 for 649 pieces of mosquito netting was warranted.[18]

Diseases that incapacitated soldiers most commonly each year of the war are shown in the following tables:

Chapter III

Table I. Leading Causes of Sickness, July 1, 1861–June 30, 1862, in all three Regions (Atlantic, Central, Pacific), called the Army of the United States, White Troops[19]

1.	Diarrhea/Dysentery	215,058
2.	Fevers	147,431
3.	Catarrh (listed with bronchitis)	83,665
4.	Rheumatism (not gout)	44,679

Troop numbers ranged between 69,118 (July 1861) and 395,713 (April 1862); mean troop strength for the year = 279,371.

Table II. Causes of Sickness, July 1, 1862–June 30, 1863, U.S. Army, White Troops[20]

1.	Diarrhea/Dysentery	521,879
2.	Fevers	339,521
3.	Rheumatism	93,307
4.	Bronchitis, acute	60,792

Troop numbers ranged between 345,010 (August 1862) to 744,780 (March 1863); mean troop strength for the year = 614,325.

Table III. Causes of Sickness, July 1, 1863–June 30, 1864, U.S. Army, White Troops[21]

1.	Diarrhea/Dysentery	395,720
2.	Fevers	384,162
3.	Rheumatism	51,953
4.	Abscess/Carbuncle/Boil	42,831

Troop numbers ranged between 567,760 (July 1863) and 696,539 (April 864); mean troop strength for the year = 619,703.

Disease Steals through the Camps

Table IV. Causes of Sickness, July 1, 1864–June 30, 1865, U.S. Army, White Troops[22]

1.	Diarrhea/Dysentery	393,783
2.	Fevers	344,558
3.	Rheumatism	56,013
4.	Abscess/Carbuncle/Boil	39,744

Troop numbers ranged between 478,268 (June 1865) to 642,008 (May 1865); mean troop strength for the year = 574,022.

Table V. Causes of Sickness, First Year after the War, July 1, 1865–June 30, 1866, U.S. Army, White Troops[23]

1.	Fevers	87,504
2.	Diarrhea/Dysentery	48,984
3.	Abscess/Boil/Carbuncle	7,852
4.	Rheumatism	7,768

Troop numbers ranged between 33,305 (May 1866) and 295,537 (July 1865); mean troop strength for the year = 99,080.

Table VI. Causes of Sickness in U.S. Colored Troops, July 1, 1863–June 30, 1864, in Atlantic and Central Regions[24]

1.	Diarrhea/Dysentery	46,572
2.	Fevers	41,921
3.	Rheumatism	9,753
4.	Bronchitis, acute	8,298

Troop numbers ranged between 12,049 (July 1863) and 71,416 (May 1864); mean troop strength for the year = 45,174.

Chapter III

Table VII. Causes of Sickness, July 1, 1864–June 30, 1865, All Regions, U.S. Colored Troops[25]

1.	Diarrhea/Dysentery	73,976
2.	Fevers	65,870
3.	Rheumatism	16,153
4.	Bronchitis, acute	7,903

Troop numbers ranged between 74,391 (September 1864) and 105,009 (June 1865); mean troop strength for the year = 89,143.

Table VIII. Causes of Sickness, July 1, 1865–June 30, 1866, All Regions, U.S. Colored Troops[26]

1.	Fevers	54,548
2.	Diarrhea/Dysentery	33,391
3.	Scurvy	7,795
4.	Rheumatism	6,219

Troop numbers ranged between 12,886 (June 1866) and 103,604 (July 1865); mean troop strength for the year = 56,617.

The burden of illness borne by soldiers reflected in these tables is truly staggering. When viewed in the context of mean troop strengths per reporting periods, many men were sick much of the time. Furthermore, the frequency with which many illnesses occurred did not lessen significantly as the war wore on. This is not surprising. Surgeons and soldiers denied insight into the roles that poor sanitation, flies and mosquitoes played in disease causation, were little able to correct these factors. Moreover, unlike the common viral diseases of childhood that resulted in immunity against future infection by those agents, the sanitation-related and mosquito-borne infections usually did not.

If the numbers of cases of the most common illnesses are impressive, deaths from them are as well. Tables IX and X show the total number of cases with the most frequently occurring sicknesses and the resulting deaths reported to the U.S. Surgeon General for the entire war.

Table IX. Leading Causes of Sickness and Resulting Deaths, July 1, 1861–June 30, 1866, U.S. Army White Troops[27]

		Ill	Dead
1.	Diarrhea/Dysentery	1,585,196	37,794
2.	Fevers	1,304,633	40,661
3.	Rheumatism	255,244	478
4.	Abscess/Boil/Carbuncle	133,009	191
5.	Scurvy	30,714	383

Table X. Leading Causes of Sickness and Resulting Deaths, July 1, 1863–June 30, 1866, U.S. Colored Troops[28]

		Ill	Dead
1.	Fevers	164,077	5,639
2.	Diarrhea/Dysentery	153,939	6,764
3.	Rheumatism	32,132	235
4.	Scurvy	16,217	388
5.	Abscess/Boil/Carbuncle	7,583	21

The monthly and quarterly reports of the sick and wounded used by the Medical Departments of both armies contained essentially the same diseases and symptoms, 137 conditions in the Union's forms,[29] and 145 in the forms of the Confederate Army.[30] Page one from *Regulations for the Army of the Confederate States* appears in Figure 1 on the next page.

Data, however, for the Confederate Army are decidedly less available. When Richmond fell in April of 1865, most of its records were destroyed. Sadly, virtually all of the writings of the South's Surgeon General, Samuel Preston Moore, were lost in the fires that consumed the city. The enormity of the lost records of just one surgeon, Joseph Jones, is alluded to by him: "At the time of the evacuation of, and destruction by fire of the government buildings in Richmond, Virginia, the manuscript volumes, containing about 1500 pages, prepared by the author, were captured or burned."[31] After the war, Dr. Jones mounted a heroic effort to reconstruct some of them. He states:

> Since the close of the war, the author has endeavored…to reproduce those portions af [sic] his labors, which appeared to be of chief interest to the Medical Profession of America, and some portions of these labors which have been brought to such a stage of completion as might admit of general conclusions, will be found in the present series of the *Medical and Surgical Memoirs*.[32]

Chapter III

CLASSES OF DISEASES.	Month,		TAKEN SICK OR RECEIVED INTO HOSPITAL DURING THE QUARTER.									
			First.		Second.		Third.		Total by each disease.		Total by each class.	
	Specific diseases.		Cases.	Deaths	Cases.	Deaths	Cases.	Deaths	Cases.	Deaths	Cases.	Deaths
Fevers	Febris Congestiva, Febris Continua Communis, Febris Intermittens Quotidiana, Febris Intermittens Tertiana, Febris Intermittens Quartana, Febris Remittens, Febris Typhoides, Febris Typhus, Febris Typhus Icterodes, All other diseases of this class,											
Eruptive fevers.	Erysipelas, Rubeola, Scarlatina, Variola, Varioloides, All other diseases of this class,											

FORM 1. *Report of the Sick and Wounded at   , for the   ending 18 .*

Figure 1. *Report of the Sick and Wounded* used by the Confederate States Army, showing the first 14 conditions listed therein. Both armies required that monthly reports on this form be forwarded eventually to their Surgeons General. Survival of these data gathered by Union surgeons allows analysis today of the diseases that plagued the armies 140 years ago. Source: S. P. Moore. Regulations of the Confederate States of America Medical Department, in *Regulations for the Army of the Confederate States*. Richmond: Randolph, 1862: 258.

Pneumonia is one disease detailed in Jones' memoirs. Like his Union counterparts, he attributes this infection to harsh climatic conditions. Pneumonia "would appear to depend in large measure upon seasons; or, in other words, upon the effects of exposure to cold and wet, and to marked vicissitudes of heat and moisture."[33] In one of Surgeon Jones' tables, covering January 1862 to July 1863, the mean strength of officers and men is 160,231; breakdown of cases is by month:

> The cases of pneumonia entered upon the Field and Hospital Reports were relatively most numerous as compared to the mean strength and the total sick and wounded during the months of December, January, February, March and April; whilst the smallest number of cases were recorded upon the field reports and transferred to the general hospitals during the months of August, September and October.[34]

Below are excerpts:

	Field reports:	**Hospital reports**
Total sick and wounded	1,057,349	397,406
Pneumonia cases	28,273	15,542 [34]

Jones reports another series occurring over fourteen months during which the Army of Tennessee experienced 8,272 cases of pneumonia, with 1,291 deaths. The hospital reports showed a still higher mortality of 18 percent.[34]

Another window into the burden of sickness suffered by the soldiers of both armies is provided in Table XIV from "Medical History," Part 3, Volume 1, of *The Medical and Surgical History of the War of the Rebellion (1861–65)* published in 1888. Direct comparison between the United States Army (USA) and the Confederate States Army (CSA), however, is not possible, since the Union cases reported here are only from the Army of the Potomac. Furthermore, these statistics include only 9 months from the Army of the Potomac, but 19 months for the Department of South Carolina, Georgia and Florida; 19 months for the Confederate forces at Mobile, Alabama; 12 months for the Department of Tennessee and 10 months for the Army of the Valley of Virginia. Nonetheless, they do allow ranking of certain diseases in order of frequency, and they do provide annual rates per thousand troop strength during the few months reported. The data in Table XI on the following page reflect the number of cases, taken directly from the above named Table XIV, reported for 9 months in the Army of the Potomac and an average of 15 months in the four Confederate armies.

These data amassed from July 1, 1861, to July 1, 1863, indicate that considerably more Confederate troops were sick from all the infections, except tonsillitis. As the Union blockade tightened and deprived the southern armies of quinine, their only effective drug against malaria, the frequency of that illness would be expected to increase even more, significantly impairing the fighting ability of the southern troops.

Henceforth, information on disease will reflect almost exclusively the views and experiences of Union surgeons and troops. *Catarrh* (the common cold) and *bronchitis* will be discussed in Chapter VI, *Abscesses/Carbuncles/Boils* in Chapter VII. *Inflammation of the lungs* (pneumonia), along with *Malaria, Dysentery/Diarrhea,* and *Typhoid Fever*, will be covered in Chapter VIII, since they were among the conditions treated with mercury during the war. *Scurvy, Diarrhea/Dysentery* and *Rheumatism* are detailed in Chapter V. The fevers that were so deadly—rheumatic fever, typhoid fever, and malaria are discussed in several locations in the book.

Soldiers who survived or avoided all of these illnesses then faced injury or death by the weapons of war, usually gunshot wounds. In fact only 7,923 cases of wounds caused by cutting (lacerations, incisions) were recorded in the Union Army during the war.[36]

To put the importance of disease during the war in perspective, one need only look at a grimmer statistic. About 4 million men were part of the war, out of a total population of 30 million counted in the census of 1860. The dead totaled more than 650,000. The cause of death in 400,000 of these young men was disease, twice the number who expired from bullets.

Table XI. Cases of Sickness and Wounds from Certain of the CSA during Portions of the Years 1861, 1862 and 1863, with the Corresponding Rates of the Army of the Potomac (USA) for nine months ending March 1862[35]

Diseases and wounds USA	151,237
Diseases and wounds CSA	495,485
Malarial fevers USA	16,781
Malarial fevers CSA	96,007
Pneumonia USA	3,233
Pneumonia CSA	11,389
Tonsillitis USA	1,312
Tonsillitis CSA	3,208
Acute bronchitis/catarrh USA	19,455
Acute bronchitis/catarrh CSA	39,345

Annual rates per thousand for these conditions:[35]

Diseases and wounds USA	2,861
Diseases and wounds CSA	4,563
Malarial fevers USA	460
Malarial fevers CSA	796
Pneumonia USA	34
Pneumonia CSA	103
Tonsillitis USA	30
Tonsillitis CSA	32
Acute bronchitis/catarrh USA	192
Acute bronchitis/catarrh CSA	415

Chapter III References

1. *Documents of the U.S. Sanitary Commission #16*, Vol. I. New York: U.S. Sanitary Commission; 1866: 1–2
2. Bayne-Jones S. *The evolution of preventive medicine in the U.S. Army, 1607–1939*. Washington: US Government Printing Office; 1968: 2
3. Steiner PE. *Disease in the Civil War*. Springfield, IL: Charles C. Thomas; 1968: 54
4. *Ibid.*, 55
5. Gershon AA. Measles Virus (Rubeola). In: Mandell GL, Bennett JE, Dolin R, eds. *Mandell, Douglas, and Bennett's Principles and Practice of Infectious Diseases*, Vol. II, 6th ed. Philadelphia: Elsevier Churchill Livingstone, Inc.; 2005: 2035
6. *Medical and Surgical History of the War of the Rebellion (1861–65)*, Part 3, Volume 1, Medical History. Washington, DC: Government Printing Office, 1888: 658. Hereafter *MSHWR (1861–1865)*
7. Shattuck L. *Report of a General Plan for the promotion of public and personal health*. Boston: Dutton and Wentworth; 1850
8. Letterman J. *Medical Recollections of the Army of the Potomac*. New York: Appleton and Co.; 1866: 98–99
9. *Ibid.*, 99
10. *Ibid.*, 100
11. *Medical and Surgical History of the War of the Rebellion (1861–65)*. Washington, DC: Government Printing Office, 1888. Repub.: *Medical and Surgical History of the Civil War*. Wilmington, NC: Broadfoot Publishing; 1990. Hereafter *MSHCW*. Vol. V; 1990: 39
12. *MSHCW* Vol. V; 1990: 42
13. *MSHWR (1861–65)*, Appendix to Part 1. 1870: 164
14. Woodward JJ. *Outlines of the Chief Camp Diseases*. Philadelphia: J.B. Lippincott & Co.; 1863: 48–50
15. *MSHWR (1861–65)*, Appendix to Part I. 1870: 78–79
16. Newberry JS. U.S.S.C. Report #36, November 30, 1861: 20–21
17. Aigner P. U.S.S.C. Report #36, November 30, 1861: 29
18. *U.S.S.C. Report #69*. New York: William C. Bryant and Co., Printers; 1863
19. *MSHWR (1861–65)*, Medical Vol. & Appendix, Part 1, Vol. 1: 146–151
20. *Ibid.*, 296–301
21. *Ibid.*, 452–457
22. *Ibid.*, 604–609
23. *Ibid.*, 630–635
24. *Ibid.*, 664–669
25. *Ibid.*, 684–689
26. *Ibid.*, 704–709
27. *Ibid.*, 636–641
28. *Ibid*, 710–712
29. *Ibid.*, 146–151
30. Moore SP. Regulations of the Confederate States of America Medical Department, in *Regulations for the Army of the Confederate States*. Richmond: Randolph; 1862. Repub.: San Francisco, Norman publishing; 1992: 258–264
31. Jones J. *Medical and Surgical Memoirs 1855–1876*, Vol. 1. New Orleans: Clark and Hofeline; 1876: preface

Chapter III

32. *Ibid.*, 651
33. *Ibid.*, 650
34. *Ibid.*, 655
35. *MSHWR (1861–65),* Medical History, Part 3, Volume 1, 1888: 32
36. *MSHWR (1861–65),* Medical History. Part 1 Volume 1, 1870: 456–457

Chapter IV.

Diarrhea and Dysentery: Bloody, but not from Bullets

During the war there were more than one and a half million officially-recorded cases of diarrhea and dysentery in U.S. White Troops[1] and over 150,000 in the U.S. Colored Troops.[2] The enormous burden these illnesses placed on an army trying to march and fight can be seen from the numbers below, especially during the first two years, when 70 to 80% of soldiers were affected with it.

Table I. Cases of Diarrhea/Dysentery per 1,000 Mean Troop Strength, All Years[1,2]

	White[1]	Colored[2]
Ending 6–30–1862	770	
Ending 6–30–1863	850	
Ending 6–30–1864	640	1060
Ending 6–30–1865	690	885
Ending 6–30–1866	494	607

The natural history of diarrhea/dysentery, especially during war, has been understood only for the past sixty years. Diarrhea is the passage of frequent watery stools that can be severe enough to cause shock and even death if the lost fluid and electrolytes (salts in body fluids) are not replaced. Dysentery is the same entity, but with bloody stools. Since the conditions that favor the two are similar, as are the infectious agents which cause them, diarrhea and dysentery are considered together here. Felsen's text of 1945 documents in detail the role of these conditions in the transmission of diarrhea and dysentery. Felsen was Director of The International and Pan-American Dysentery Registry. Ingestion of food or water contaminated by fecal matter containing certain strains of rod-shaped (bacilli) bacteria—*Shigella* or *Salmonella*, but not the *Salmonella* that causes typhoid fever—result in "food poisoning," with diarrhea or dysentery. Patients recovering from these infections "usually excrete the...[bacteria] for...seven to ten days. The greatest danger in bacillary dysentery is from...carriers...[with] chronic...dysentery, or from mild and unrecognized acute (sudden onset, rapid resolution) forms of the disease."[3]

Not until fifty years after the Civil War was the crucial role played by flies in spreading these diseases recognized. Dysentery is "most prevalent when the fly population is at its

Chapter IV

maximum. This is particularly true...where sanitation is poor."[4] Dysentery follows about ten days after climatic conditions become favorable for the breeding of flies. "With the onset of severe frost the flies are paralyzed and [then] sporadic cases occur due to human factors [such as infected feces on unwashed hands]."[4] In 1912 and 1913 houseflies also were proven to carry the bacteria that cause dysentery, contaminating food by vomiting or defecating on it after feeding on dysenteric stools.[4] *Shigella* organisms were "actually isolated from the intestinal tracts of two houseflies caught on the bed of a dysentery patient."[4] Bacteria could be recovered five days after flies were seen feeding. Dysentery bacteria were shown to survive in the intestinal tract of the fly three days after being ingested.[4] Flies that fed on milk or on dried feces remained infective for 24 hours.[4]

Although these studies show that the intestinal tract is a "source of dysentery organisms in infected flies, ...the hairs...of the legs contaminated by contact with infected material are probably the most common conveyers of the bacteria to food."[4] Felsen describes the life cycle of the housefly with its potential to generate prodigious numbers of progeny:

> In warm weather, the larvae or maggots hatch out in a few hours to become pupae and in about five days longer, adult insects. It has been estimated that one egg-laying female can give rise in six months to more than 131 quintillions [131×10^{18}] of descendants, if all eggs laid came to maturity. It has also been calculated that one fly, after feeding on the contents of a spitoon [sic] or manure pile, can carry 500 to 6 million bacteria on its body.[5]

Milk can be a source of infection, especially via food handlers. "Under experimental conditions, sterile...milk inoculated with...strains...[of *Shigella* which can cause dysentery] and kept at room temperature revealed the persistence of viable...[bacteria] for two to six months."[6]

Water from contaminated wells is often a vehicle of transmission. Experiments reveal that the dysentery organism can survive in water for four weeks after the inoculation of sterile water and six weeks after the inoculation of tap water with this bacterium.[7] A 1918 study showed that organisms causing *Shigella* dysentery survived, and actually increased "in stored water, especially at low or medium temperature. Chlorination was incapable of rendering contaminated water safe, but the dysentery organisms were destroyed quickly by the direct action of sun rays."[7]

Abundant evidence that flies and exposed feces existed during the Civil War was documented in the previous chapter. Without hand washing as recognized prophylaxis against ingestion of fecal matter, there is little doubt that unsanitary food and fingers figured in the spread of diarrhea and dysentery.

One hundred years after the Civil War an epidemic of *Shigella*-induced diarrhea occurred aboard a U.S. Naval ship, documenting the threat to armed forces that it still poses. This outbreak happened while the ship was in port in an area endemic for *Shigella*. Two cooks meticulously prepared a picnic. The medical report indicates that:

> Elaborate sanitary precautions were taken by the food-handlers, who were well aware of the hazards inherent in large picnics. Meats were prepared whole, wrapped, refrigerated until actually required, and sliced just before serving. Salads were mixed as required, instead of being prepared in advance.

Even the bread was sliced only just before being placed on the serving line. [Unfortunately, the food handlers had dysentery they were trying to hide, and failed to wash their hands while preparing the food.] [They] had contracted dysentery ashore, and were mildly ill. [They] took great pains to conceal their infirmities, because they feared that they might be hospitalized and so lose their promised liberty at the conclusion of the picnic—and it was the ship's last night in port. Consequently, their work of preparing food for service upon the cafeteria-style serving line was interspersed by repeated hurried trips to the toilet. They dared not take time for hand washing lest their absences be noted. It must be presumed, therefore, that much of the food these cooks prepared became contaminated.[8]

Much of the diarrhea and dysentery during the Civil War could have been prevented had the surgeons known the procedures set forth by Felsen in 1945: immediate isolation of any men with diarrhea; burial and oil treatment of all excreta; adequate screening against, and destruction of, flies; sterilization of contaminated material by boiling; immediate relief from duty for food handlers with diarrhea; boiling of all food; and boiling of water.[9] Alas, doctors of the Civil War did not know of these simple interventions.

In most victims of diarrhea/dysentery who survive, the illness runs a course of several days to several weeks and engenders no complications other than dehydration and the loss of certain chemicals from the body. In some patients, however, there is an immune reaction one week to one month later which leads to one or more of these complications: sudden painful swelling in several joints; genital and skin rashes; a severe form of arthritis involving the spine (ankylosing spondylitis); conjunctivitis or even involvement of the iris of the eye which may result in blindness. These complications of diarrhea or dysentery imposed additional miseries on armies already debilitated, as the next chapter will document.

Chapter IV References

1. *Medical and Surgical History of the War of the Rebellion (1861–65)*. Washington, DC: Government Printing Office, 1888, Medical Vol. & Appendix, Part 1, Vol. 1: 636
2. *Ibid.*, 710
3. Felsen J. *Bacillary Dysentery Colitis and Enteritis*. Philadelphia: W.B. Saunders Co.; 1945: 46
4. *Ibid.*, 52
5. *Ibid.*, 288
6. *Ibid.*, 56
7. *Ibid.*, 57
8. Noer HR. An "experimental" epidemic of Reiter's Syndrome. *JAMA*. 1966; 198: 693–698
9. Felsen J. *Bacillary Dysentery Colitis and Enteritis*. Philadelphia: W.B. Saunders Co.; 1945: 288–289

Chapter V.

Rheumatism: Soldiers in Bed, not in Battle

Several medical scholars of the Civil War have noted that rheumatism figured prominently in the war. Steiner refers to rheumatism as an old military pest and "sometimes a sequel of infection."[1] In August and September of 1861, when Robert E. Lee was trying to bring western Virginia under Confederate control (western Virginia did not secede from the Union as did Virginia), rheumatism was one of the conditions that so enervated his troops that he withdrew them without having fought at all.[2] Similarly, McClellan's 1861 western Virginia campaign was severely deterred, "dysentery, diarrhea, malaria, typhoid fever, measles, and rheumatism…taking out over 20,000 men from July to October, [and] rendering many regiments wholly unfit for duty."[3]

Regarding the Peninsular Campaign of 1862, Steiner points out that:

> Acute and chronic rheumatism were a major problem in camp and field, especially during the winter months. This disease decreased in April 1862, but in June there was a sharp rise. This may represent proximity to the battlefields of the Peninsula rather than a true increase because this was a favorite complaint with malingerers. In nine months, 15,517 cases and five deaths were recorded. This diagnosis included what today would be called variously rheumatic fever, rheumatoid arthritis, osteoarthritis, the arthritis of specific infections (gonococcal, tuberculous, etc.), and other diseases. Some of the gouty arthritis was probably included, although thirty-six cases of gout were separately reported under this diagnosis.[4]

In the first campaign for Corinth, Mississippi (May of 1862), in the Department of the Tennessee (U.S.A.), the data from some of Halleck's men show rheumatism to be one of their largest problems. There were 2,250 examples, including 1,301 of the acute and 949 of the chronic forms. This diagnosis included rheumatic fever and other diseases.[5] In the Confederate States Army chronic rheumatism was one reason for discharge of 13 members of Company F of the 21st Virginia during the War. In this same company 26 died in combat, 24 were captured, and 27 wounded, of whom 9 were discharged because of a wound. Three died of disease.[6]

Of the health of Union soldiers in Washington, D.C., Freemon comments, "The more common diseases among the Washington troops were diarrhea, typhoid fever, rheumatism, malaria, measles, and venereal disease."[7]

Finally, Freemon quotes a letter written late in the war (April 26, 1864) by Walt Whitman, who gave comfort and aid to injured or ill soldiers "The number of sick are 'becoming alarmingly greater,' suffering from 'diarrhea, rheumatism, and the old camp fevers.' "[8]

A detailed look at the importance of rheumatism in the war. In the *Sickness and Mortality Reports of White Troops* from the *Medical and Surgical History of the War of the Rebellion (1861–1865)* "Rheumatism" was the fourth most frequent diagnosis the first year of the war. In the second year it rose to third place, after "Diarrhea/ Dysentery" and "Fevers," where it remained throughout the conflict.[9] The United States Colored Troops (U.S.C.T) were similarly affected.[10] In 254,738 cases of rheumatism in white soldiers, there were 475 deaths;[11] in 32,125 cases in U.S.C.T., there occurred 235 deaths.[12] Of all white troops who acquired a rheumatic disease, 4.6% were discharged with disability;[13] the comparable percentage in U.S.C.T. was 2.7%.[14] Detailed statistics appear in Tables I through VIII in Chapter III. These are summarized in the table below:

Table I. Cases of Rheumatism per 1,000 Mean Troop Strength, all years of the War

	White	Colored
Ending 6–30–1862	160	
Ending 6–30–1863	152	
Ending 6–30–1864	84	215
Ending 6–30–1865	98	181
Ending 6–30–1866	78	110

Definitions of rheumatism and rheumatic disease. A very old term, *rheumatism* connotes pain, stiffness, and limited motion of joints because of disease arising in joints themselves or in muscles, tendons, ligaments or bones attached to them. As recently as 1987, the American College of Rheumatology (founded in 1934 by physicians in the United States who specialized in the care of patients with arthritis, osteoporosis, and other diseases of the muscles and skeleton) was called the American Rheumatism Association. *Arthritis* is a very specific term that denotes swelling, pain, warmth, and variable redness in a joint, with resulting loss of the ability to fully bend, straighten or rotate the joint. *Rheumatic disease* applies to structures other than merely the joints, e.g., tendons, bursas, muscles. Presently more than 100 distinct types of rheumatic disease are recognized.

Considerable guesswork is involved in categorizing the rheumatic diseases represented in Civil War case reports because surgeons' descriptions are few and sketchy, and because a given patient may be suffering from more than one disease or entity at the same time. Several allusions to rheumatic diseases, usually without details, by a dozen physicians serving in the war or on the U.S. Sanitary Commission also survive. Clearly these diseases impaired the marching and fighting capacity of the Union Army. Unfortunately, no such records survive from the Confederate Army, since they were destroyed when Richmond was burned. Despite the large number of cases of rheumatism reported by the Union Army (286,863, including gout),[11,12] the *Medical and Surgical History of the War of the Rebellion (1861–1865)* details only 44 patients with rheumatic diseases. Even so, these few case reports do provide valuable information. Cared for in 23 hospitals in 11 states, these soldiers' diseases will now be analyzed.

Surgeons distinguished between "acute" and "chronic" rheumatism not only in the required *monthly reports* to the Medical Director and in *quarterly reports* to the Surgeon General of the Union Army, but also in *case reports* describing features of these diseases. Thirteen case reports are designated "acute" rheumatism.[14] These are defined as having a duration of joint pain and swelling for one week or less (4 patients), two to four weeks (6 patients), and longer than four months (3 cases). In soldiers with "chronic" rheumatism painful swelling in joints persisted for two to four weeks in 1 patient, three months or less in 7, four to six months in 8, seven to twelve months in 7, longer than one year in 6, and longer than five years in 1; in one case report the duration of rheumatism is not given.[15] Because "acute" and "chronic" are never defined, and because of overlap in the duration of symptoms between the groups, the distinction appears arbitrary and useless. Patients, therefore, are considered in this chapter as a single group, having *rheumatic disease,* or *rheumatism*. These limitations notwithstanding, there appears to be at least eleven types of rheumatic disease that affected soldiers serving in the war:

1. Rheumatic fever
2. Arthritis following dysentery/diarrhea or after non-gonorrheal urethritis (reactive arthritis)
3. Serious spine inflammation (ankylosing spondylitis)
4. Scurvy (scorbutic arthritis)
5. Tuberculosis
6. Septic arthritis (pus in a joint), with or without a wound
7. Gonococcal (gonorrheal) arthritis, two patterns
8. Syphilis
9. Rheumatoid arthritis
10. Malaria
11. Gout
12. Mumps

1. Rheumatic fever. This disease has been the scourge of men in armies throughout history, until cots were arranged in head-toe alternation in their quarters, and penicillin prophylaxis and treatment of streptococcal throat infections was begun. This did not occur until World War II—until the cause of rheumatic fever was known to be an abnormal immune response in a patient whose throat was infected by a particular streptococcus (Group A), until crowding of recruits was understood to facilitate droplet spread of the bacterium, until it was recognized that certain critical numbers of streptococcal sore throats (pharyngitis) were associated with development of rheumatic fever, and until penicillin was available and used to treat Group A streptococcal throat infections without symptoms as well as those with pain. That's a number of "untils"!

Clinical picture and diagnosis. Rheumatic fever involves the heart and has an associated arthritis, a characteristic skin rash, nodules in the skin, uncoordinated jerking movements of the arms and legs (chorea) and a sore throat, first described by Cheadle in 1889.[16] Criteria that allow us to define this disease were developed by T. Duckett Jones in 1944.[17] Jones' Criteria included any combination of Major Criteria or one Major and two Minor Criteria, as shown in the table on the next page:

Table II. Jones Criteria for Diagnosis of Rheumatic Fever, 1944[17]

Major	Minor
Carditis	Fever
Arthralgia	Precordial (chest) pain
Chorea	Erythema marginatum
Nodules	Nosebleed
Previous rheumatic fever	Anti-Streptolysin O (ASO) titer
	Throat culture positive for Group A streptococcus

The occurrence of abdominal pain, chest pain, "pulmonary changes," and nosebleed in conditions other than rheumatic fever caused them to be dropped as diagnostic indicators. Further scientific understanding in the latter half of the twentieth century led to other modifications in the criteria, such that the most recent formulation in 1992 is seen below:

Table III. Diagnostic Criteria for Rheumatic Fever, 1992[18]

Major	Minor
Carditis	Fever
Polyarthritis	Elevated acute phase reactants
Chorea	Prolonged PR interval on EKG
Nodules	ASO Titer or other anti-streptococcal blood test
Erythema marginatum	Throat culture positive for Group A streptococcus

A diagnosis of rheumatic fever now requires a patient to have two major, or one major and two minor, criteria plus evidence of a prior Group A streptococcal infection (" strep throat"). **Definitions:** *Acute phase reactants* are chemicals present in the blood when an infection is present; they are not detectable when the infection either has run its course or responds to treatment. Anti-Streptolysin O (ASO) titer is a blood test indicating a recent infection with a bacterium, the streptococcus. A *throat culture* is done by placing material obtained from the throat of a person suspected of having a streptococcal infection on a sterile glass dish filled with gelatin. There are many types of streptococci, but only one, Group A, causes rheumatic fever. The type of streptococcus can be identified after it grows on the sterile (Petri) dish. A *prolonged PR interval*, commonly found in rheumatic fever, results in a heartbeat that is not normal. It is diagnosed using an instrument called an electrocardiograph.

Manifestations of rheumatic fever, such as chorea or erythema marginatum will be defined as they are encountered in the case reports.

A patient with a "strep throat" is feverish, with pain, swelling and redness of the pharynx. The tonsils are also "enlarged and reddened" and covered, in Krause's words, with "yellow-gray" pus.[19] See Figure 1.

Krause summarizes our present understanding of how strep throats are spread:

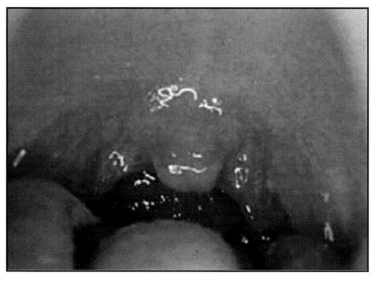

Figure 1. Strep throat (infection of the throat or tonsils with Group A streptococcus) results, two to four weeks later, in acute rheumatic fever in 3% of untreated cases. *Photograph courtesy of J. Santoro, M.D.*

> Transmission occurs as a result of close contact between susceptible individuals and other infected persons or healthy individuals who carry contagious streptococci in the pharynx. Organisms are transmitted from one person to another on saliva droplets...[ejected] by sneezing or coughing. For this reason, transmission of this disease requires close association with an individual who harbors infectious streptococci in the pharynx.[19]

Approximately 3% of people with Group A streptococcal infection of the throat who are not treated will develop rheumatic fever.[20]

A patient with rheumatic fever has fever and joint pain, with or without swelling. If unaccompanied by swelling, it is called *arthralgia*; if swelling of the joints is present, *arthritis*. The pain is excruciating, making the patient unable to turn over in bed, get out of bed, or feed himself. Characteristically the pain moves from one joint to another, persisting several hours in a knee, for example, before moving to a shoulder or wrist. According to Bisno, as many as 16 joints may be involved in an episode of rheumatic fever, and six or more joints are commonly affected.[21] The joint pain is dramatically relieved by aspirin, but this was not used widely until 1898, nearly forty years after the Civil War.

The third most common feature, and the dangerous one, is heart involvement. If the outer covering of the heart (pericardium) is involved, the patient has chest pain as the pericardium stretches with the pumping action of the heart or touches the inner rib cage. Corresponding to this friction is a "friction rub," often heard with the stethoscope. If heart valves (endocarditis) are affected, blood from the lungs may not be able to be emptied from the lungs to enter the left side of the heart, causing shortness of breath; fluid may back up if the right side of the heart cannot admit and retain blood, accumulating in the legs or abdomen, causing "dropsy;" or blood may not be able to enter the circulation because the aortic valve is too tightly scarred, causing unconsciousness or death. Furthermore, valves that have been damaged and become misshapen can trap bacteria that may be present in the bloodstream and result in death by infection (bacterial endocarditis). The most catastrophic

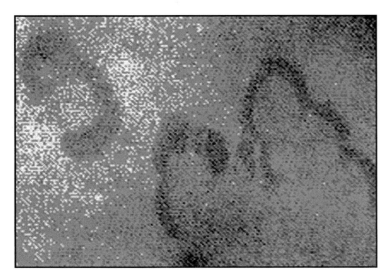

Figure 2. "Smoke rings" of erythema marginatum skin rash. *Author's collection.*

consequence, however, of rheumatic fever involving the heart is impairment of the pumping action because of damage to the heart muscle itself (myocarditis). Death occurs quickly because of sudden heart failure; the patient essentially drowns and suffocates. Civil War surgeons would not have been able to suspect the diagnosis with an EKG (electrocardiogram), since this was not in use until 1903.[22] Without diuretics, they would not have been able to treat heart failure effectively, even if recognized.

The nodules and erythema marginatum rash are uncommon and often difficult to detect. Nodules occur on elbows or the back of the head, where a sick patient or a busy surgeon would probably not look. The rash is evanescent, like pink smoke rings (shown in Figure 2), on the trunk and abdomen, areas usually covered by clothing. In men who had to be forced to change clothing or bathe once a week, a non-itchy, non-painful rash or painless nodules could have been overlooked easily by the patient. Chorea, first described by Thomas Sydenham,[23] is rare and is not seen during the episode of fever, joint pain or cardiac involvement, but occurs many months later. Hence it would have been unlikely that surgeons caring for acutely ill soldiers would link chorea and rheumatic fever. Chorea, also called St. Vitus' Dance, was diagnosed during the Civil War as an entity,[24] but not recognized as a manifestation of rheumatic fever. The immune studies required to establish the diagnosis today, e.g., Anti-Streptolysin O Titer, reflect twentieth century advances in immunology and microbiology which have taught us about the complicated ability of certain streptococci to cause human disease, and could not have been used during the Civil War.

Civil War cases that might be rheumatic fever. Knowing whether rheumatic diseases were indeed cases of rheumatic fever in the Civil War is exceedingly difficult because of often sketchy descriptions of cases and because sore throat was rarely mentioned. Since there is a two to four week interval between the sore throat and the heart or joint complaints, probably neither patient nor surgeon would connect the two events. These shortcomings notwithstanding, of the 44 cases of rheumatism recorded in the *Medical and Surgical History of the War of the Rebellion (1861–1865),*[25] fifteen have features consistent with rheumatic fever. Nine of these appear below, with commentary. Details of cases are written in the staccato, terse style of the reporting surgeon.

Case 1. P.H., no age given. Admitted 1-24-1862 with back pain and sore swollen ankles; left knee involved too, but not described, duration unknown. Pulse elevated, hot skin. Pain disturbed sleep. 24 hours later ankles still very painful, although only slightly swollen, "but right knee hot, swollen and painful; pulse accelerated; skin hot." At 48 hours "both knees hot and...swollen, but the right only painful; ankles sound...; pulse 80." Three days after admission "pain only in the left knee, which is enlarged from effusion [fluid in the joint]; pulse about 60, very irregular; skin hot; pain in the region of the heart. Five days after admission rested well; appears well; pulse regular...." Discharged 6th day to quarters. Treated with colchicum. Duration of rheumatic symptoms: 6 days (?). *Hospital 28th Mass.*[26]

Comment. Although thermometers were known at the time of the Civil War, body temperature of patients is almost never recorded. As in this case, skin of patients with fever is usually simply described as "hot." The migratory pattern of the arthritis in rheumatic fever is illustrated in this patient, as the swelling subsided in his ankles, and moved to his knees. "Pain in the region of the heart" was probably pericarditis.

Case 6. J.R., age 20. Admitted 9–23–1863 with chest pain, cough, coughing up "occasional" blood. Feb. 3, 1864, "attacked with acute rheumatism, the knee-joints...painful and swollen. On the 5th, as...knees improved, his feet and ankles became swollen and he was seized with cardiac pain and...[difficulty breathing], while friction sounds were heard on auscultation. These symptoms continued with increasing gravity and much restlessness, and on the 11th the friction sounds were obscured by pericardial effusion. He gradually sank, and died on the 26th." Autopsy: lungs compressed, right lung dense, stuck to diaphragm, left lung lining stuck to pericardium; pericardium thickened and "distended with 40 ounces of turbid" fluid. Duration of symptoms: 23 days. *Cumberland Hospital, Md.*[27]

Comment. "Friction sounds" are heard with the help of a stethoscope and are typical of pericarditis, common in rheumatic fever. There are numerous references to heart and lung sounds detected by this instrument. John Ordronaux lists the stethoscope, along with a watch "to test deafness, pulse, breathing," magnifying glass "to examine the eyes and cutaneous diseases," spatula (presumably tongue depressor), measuring tape, urethral catheter and sound, laryngoscope, speculum (instrument to permit visualizaiton of a body opening) for the ear and for the anus/rectum, and ophthalmoscope, as equipment needed by a surgeon.[28]

Case 8. J.B., no age given. Admitted 3–19–1865 with "rheumatic fever." No mention of joints at all. On 4–4 diarrhea and "gastric irritation." On 4–6 difficulty breathing, "tumultuous" action of the heart, heart enlargement by dullness to percussion, irregular, "small" pulse. *Died* on 4–8. Autopsy: thick pericardium containing 6 ounces of fluid, clots in both ventricles. Duration of symptoms: 3 weeks "fever;" joints unknown. *Harewood Hospital, Washington, D.C.*[27]

Comment. The enlarged heart was probably caused by fluid in the pericardium. The "tumultuous" action reflected irregularity of the pulse, common in rheumatic fever. The "small" pulse was due to constriction of the heart by fluid trapped in the pericardium, restricting the amount of blood the heart could eject into the circulation. Now, high doses of cortisone and surgical drainage of the pericardial fluid would prevent a soldier's death from this complication.

Case 9. W.P.T., age 24. Admitted 12-2-1863 "with diphtheria. He was improving under quinine and chlorate of potash internally, ...alternating with nitrate of silver, as a local application when he was attacked with acute rheumatism, the knees and elbows being specially affected. He stated that he had been subject to attacks of this kind all his life." No further details given. Seemed to recover until 12-22, when "seized with sharp cutting pains in the bladder and side, and died half an hour afterwards." Treated with saline cathartics also. Autopsy: "An enormous pericardial effusion [accumulation of fluid in the sac that surrounds the heart] with some adhesions was found...." No mention of an abdominal examination. Duration of symptoms: 2 weeks (?). *Jarvis Hospital, Baltimore Md.*[27]

Comment. This soldier probably had rheumatic fever during childhood, with characteristic arthritis and heart involvement after each subsequent streptococcal sore throat. It is well known that people who have had rheumatic fever "have...abnormal reactivity to group A streptococcal infections. Recurrent rheumatic fever develops in 40% to 50% of such persons if they have a streptococcal infection during the first year after the initial episode of rheumatic fever. As years pass without recurrences of rheumatic fever, ...[the tendency to have another episode] wanes, but the probability of recurrence does not entirely disappear."[29] Major Charles Smart, who succeeded Joseph Janvier Woodward as author of the third part of the *MSHWR* of 1888, wrote that in recurrent rheumatism:

> A majority of the...men affected were known...to have suffered...from the disease before their enlistment. On exposure they became temporarily crippled. Under favorable conditions they so far recovered as to be able to resume duty, but on a subsequent exposure they were again taken on the sick report....[30]

Some types of arthritis prevented a man from being accepted into the army, e.g. tuberculosis of the spine and joints with chronic swelling and deformity.[31] The arthritis of rheumatic fever, however, does not leave deformities in its wake; when the episode has run its course, the joints return to their normal pre-attack appearance. Thus a man with previous rheumatic fever would not have been rejected from the service. The "diphtheria" in Case 9 may instead have been streptococcal pharyngitis, the necessary antecedent to rheumatic fever. Growing bacteria in the laboratory to distinguish the diphtheria bacterium from the streptococcus would not be possible until Robert Koch's work of the 1870s.

Case 12. E.M.D., age 20. Admitted 10-5-1864 "with...disease of the heart." Suffered "a short time before" from "an attack of articular rheumatism." He had fluid in the abdomen, shortness of breath, "rapid and tumultuous action of the heart unaccompanied by any decided bellows murmur...." He "preferred the sitting posture." More irregular pulse, more trouble breathing. Died 10-7. Autopsy: Fluid around right lung, congested lungs, greatly dilated heart, only 2 ounces of fluid in pericardium; "small, firm, wart-like excrescences were found on the mitral valve and large ones on the aortic valves...." Duration of symptoms: 1 week (?). *Carver Hospital, Washington, D.C.*[32]

Chapter V

> **Case 37**. C.B., age 34. Admitted 3–25–1865, "chronic rheumatism and heart disease." Onset or further details not given. "Great" trouble breathing and "heart sounds…obscured by a…murmur;" died "suddenly" 5–27–1865. Autopsy: "The pericardium was closely and firmly adherent to the heart, which was very large, weighing thirty ounces; the mitral and semilunar [aortic] valves were thickened and covered with warty vegetations." Duration of rheumatic symptoms: more than 2 months (?). *Jarvis Hospital, Baltimore, Md.*[33]

Comment. The "wart-like" growths on the heart valves in the last two cases illustrate a complication of rheumatic fever, namely, seeding of previously damaged valves by bacteria that enter the bloodstream, called bacterial endocarditis.

> **Case 14**. J.L.W., age 38. Admitted 9–28–1863, rheumatic fever followed by 4 weeks of rheumatic pains. Able to walk 10–14; returned to duty 10–19–1863. Duration of rheumatic symptoms: 3 weeks. Mustered out 6–7–1865. *Officers' Hospital, Louisville, Ky.*[34]

Comment. This soldier's arthritis is typical of rheumatic fever. Although the course of the untreated disease is three months, the arthritis subsides in three weeks. He may not have had heart involvement, or experienced such mild cardiac disease that he would have been able to return to duty without limitation of activity.

> **Case 31**. J.F.S., age 21. Admitted 5–7–1863, after rheumatism, approximately 10–1862. Surgeon found high pulse (106 beats per minute), "jerking" heart impulse; patient had "pain on exertion," severe "shooting pains in joints, hips and various parts of the body." By 8–17–1863 "recovered except swelling of right hand", but 8–20 "rheumatism passed to other joints." Discharged 8–21–1863. Duration of rheumatic symptoms: 10 months. *Satterlee Hospital, Philadelphia, Pa.*[35]

Comment. He may have had recurrent episodes of rheumatic fever, but the history is too vague to establish this with certainty.

> **Case 32**. J.M., age 28. Admitted 12–8–1864, after rheumatism "mostly in the knees" 11–1864; surgeon found shortness of breath on exertion, pulse 120, increased heart impulse; patient had left chest pain. By 1–1–1865 pulse "still rapid; dyspnoea [shortness of breath] aggravated; countenance livid." No better by 3–29–1865; discharged. Duration of rheumatic symptoms: 4 months. *Hospital, Quincy, Ill.*[35]

Comment. Note that the soldiers' ages ranged between 20 and 40 years in these cases. Most initial attacks of rheumatic fever in adults "take place at the end of the second and beginning of the third decades of life. Rarely, initial attacks occur as late as the fourth decade and recurrent attacks have been documented as late as the fourth decade."[20]

Historical experience with rheumatic fever in the armed forces. During World War II and the Korean War epidemic streptococcal throat infections and rheumatic fever were common. As Heggie notes, Group A streptococcal infections are numerous where:

> Large numbers of persons live and work in close proximity and where there is a rapid turnover of personnel. Navy and Marine Corps [and Army] recruit populations fall into this category. Accordingly, ...[Group A streptococcal] pharyngitis and its complication, ...[rheumatic fever] have been important problems in these groups. For example, during World War II, 21,209 cases of...[rheumatic fever] occurred in Navy and Marine Corps recruits between 1942 and 1945.[36]

The number of cases at the Naval Training Center in Farragut, Idaho, was so high and so continuous that recruit training there was terminated in 1944.[36] In 1951 a streptococcal control program was begun in Navy and Marine Corps training centers, which consisted of:

- Weekly counts of cases of Group A streptococcal pharyngitis year-round

- Injection of long-acting penicillin on the 14th day of training to incoming recruits from October to April, except at Orlando, Florida (where a very low number of cases of strep throat occurred)

- Repeat penicillin injection on 42nd day of training (duration of training is 8 weeks) if Group A streptococcal sore throats exceed 10 cases per 1,000 recruits per week at or beyond the 42nd training day

- Penicillin prophylaxis, regardless of month of the year or location, if Group A streptococcal pharyngitis equals or exceeds 10 cases per 1,000 recruits per week, continuing for 6 weeks or until Group A streptococcal sore throats drop below 10 cases per 1,000 recruits per week. Excluded are penicillin-allergic recruits; Group A streptococcal infections in this group are treated with 10 days of erythromycin.[36]

Training centers discontinued this program after rheumatic fever declined markedly. The disease has reappeared periodically since the cessation of routine penicillin prophylaxis. In June of 1968, six cases of rheumatic fever occurred at Lowry Air Force Base, Colorado, the first in 10 years at that facility.[37] In 1986 and 1987, ten cases occurred at the Navy Training Center in San Diego, the first outbreak there in over 20 years.[38] The patients were 19 to 31 years of age:

> During this outbreak the mean time from entering training to diagnosis and hospitalization was 44 days. This finding is consistent with past experience and with current Navy streptococcal infection control directives, which suggest that medical departments be especially aware of the potential occurrence of...[rheumatic fever] about 42 days after training begins. Mass prophylaxis with Benzathine penicillin G has been reinstituted at...[the Navy Training Center].[38]

One year later 14 cases of rheumatic fever occurred among Army trainees at Fort Leonard Wood, Missouri. Like patients with rheumatic fever throughout history, they manifest the disease with carditis (heart inflammation) (8 cases), arthritis involving several joints (12), erythema marginatum (1) and subcutaneous nodules (1):

> An investigation based on data from routine hospital surveillance showed that hospitalization rates for acute respiratory disease…had also increased during the fall of 1987 among personnel in basic training.… A review of…throat cultures obtained from these patients indicated that recovery of…Group A streptococci increased from approximately 25% in late summer to more than 79% in early fall…[38]

In contrast, there were no cases of rheumatic fever in civilians reported in neighboring hospitals or by the respective health departments during this period.[38]

Evidence that conditions existed during the Civil War favoring development of rheumatic fever. It is well established that crowding is associated with individual attacks, and especially with outbreaks, of acute rheumatic fever.[20] There is abundant documentation that close living quarters were common during the war. Olmstead, in U.S. Sanitary Commission Report #40 (12-9-1861), wrote of the Army of the Potomac:

> Six men are usually provided with lodging in one of the 'wedge' tents. In the Sibley tent from twelve to sixteen; of late sometimes twenty. [The men] burrow or seal themselves in their lodgings [in anticipation of winter; there is a] natural disposition of soldiers to shut themselves up in their tents or huts as much and as closely as possible in cold weather. In many camps they…[are] already…excavating the ground within their lodgings, and throwing up banks of earth against their walls or curtains. This practice…should at once be forbidden, and full ventilation of tents at night made compulsory.…[39]

The tendency of streptococcal sore throats to increase in the autumn and winter is reflected in the rheumatic fever prophylaxis guidelines of 1951, above, which required all recruits to be given penicillin between October and April. Ninety years before, Olmstead noted "a slight but appreciable increase in cases of disease appropriate to the winter months, as severe colds, …pulmonary affections, and *acute rheumatism* [emphasis added]."[39] Olmstead's observation is important, since we know that sneezing and coughing spread the Group A streptococcus. Presumably sore throat (pharyngitis) not accompanied by symptoms of a cold also increased in winter, since their mechanism of transmission is the same, but Civil War surgeons did not use "pharyngitis." They did use "cynanche" for sore throat, but the *Sickness and Mortality Reports* contain neither word; "inflammation of the tonsils," or *tonsillitis* in modern parlance, would seem to be the closest relevant term. If *tonsillitis* is used as a surrogate for *pharyngitis*, there is a rise in the late fall and winter among soldiers in the Civil War, shown in Tables I through VIII in Appendix III. In all years of the war, in white as well as colored troops, tonsillitis peaked between December and March, paralleling the increase observed in recruits in World War II.

One might then expect an increase in cardiac disease two to four weeks later, i.e., January through April, since rheumatic fever follows streptococcal pharyngitis by that interval. Cases of heart disease in the Civil War were comprised of five categories—*inflammation of the endocardium, inflammation of the pericardium, dropsy from heart disease, dropsy of the pericardium*, and *valvular disease of the heart*—when recorded in the *Sickness and Mortality Reports*. Tables IX through XVI, in Appendix III, show the number of cases of cardiac disease in each month of the war.

In these tables, however, we see peak occurrences of cardiac disease in months other than January through April—in October, November, and July. This doesn't mean that rheumatic fever was not present, but probably that heart disease is more complicated to diagnose than tonsillitis or pharyngitis, especially with limited use of a stethoscope and no availability of electrocardiography or echocardiography. Also data would undercount mild cases of carditis (few or no symptoms) that may have begun in January through April and would record these as having occurred several weeks after the onset of actual heart involvement in indolent cases. Furthermore, since one-third of Group A streptococcal throat infections may be silent (detected since 1932 by elevated Anti-Streptolysin O Titers in the blood, verifying the antecedent infection responsible for the heart damage), patients could have contracted "strep throat" without symptoms in a non-epidemic setting, e.g., in September, October, or June, and reported to the surgeon in October, November or July, respectively.

Alternatively, other causes of heart disease, e.g., endocarditis or diphtheria, which do not necessarily have a predilection to cluster in cold weather, could be the causative agent. The former is caused by bacteria in the bloodstream that lodge on the heart valves, grow there, and destroy them. In diphtheria the bacterium causing the disease produces a toxin which causes the heart muscle to fail, causing irregular heartbeat, collapse of the circulation and congestive heart failure, as seen in rheumatic fever; nasal or oral droplet spread, or skin lesions, spread the highly contagious disease. We know that endocarditis and diphtheria occurred during the Civil War and that surgeons of the time recognized these entities. In Cases 12 and 37 under *Civil War Cases that might be Rheumatic Fever*, above, endocarditis is described at post-mortem. Diphtheria, with its typical tightly adherent membrane covering the throat, is well described in 26 cases, all of them autopsied, in the *MSHWR*.[40]

Mortality. Tonsillitis resulted in death in 0.08 to 0.2% of white troops and 0.1 to 0.2% of colored troops, shown in Tables I through VIII in Appendix III, probably as a result of peritonsillar abscess, pneumonia, or infection of the pleural space. Death rates from heart disease, Tables IX through XVI, varied from 16 to 18% in white troops and tragically from 38 to 61% in colored troops. Mortality from rheumatic fever is not known to have a racial predisposition, unless accompanied by economic disadvantage and its consequent crowded living.

Discharge with disability was granted because of heart disease in 10,859 of the 215,312 white soldiers disabled for all reasons, accounting for 5% of discharges with disability.[41] For the U.S. Colored Troops, the corresponding numbers were 174 men of 8,223 disabled, or 2% of all discharges with disability.[42]

Summary. Close living quarters inherent in times of war are associated with easy transmission of bacteria that inhabit the throat and respiratory tract. One such bacterium, the Group A streptococcus, is especially dangerous, because in certain people the infection will result in rheumatic fever. The fever and painful joint swelling are disabling for a few weeks, but heart involvement may persist for months, become sufficiently severe or chronic to eventuate in discharge from military service, or prove fatal. Once rheumatic fever develops in an individual, it occurs again with each new streptococcal throat infection. Since there was no effective treatment during the Civil War, we are able to see the natural history of this serious rheumatic disease and sympathize with the many young men who suffered its consequences.

2. Arthritis following dysentery/ diarrhea or after non-gonorrheal urethritis (reactive arthritis). Chapter IV detailed the frequency with which dysentery and diarrhea occurred in the war, how the lack of recognition that food, feces, flies and fingers were responsible for their spread promoted recurrent outbreaks and the development in a few soldiers of arthritis as a complication. Consideration will now be given to those in whom the intestinal infection is followed by an immune reaction one week to one month later—leading to sudden painful swelling in several joints, to genital and skin rashes, and to conjunctivitis and even involvement of the iris of the eye with blindness. The same abnormal immune response to the rod-shaped bacteria causing dysentery/ diarrhea occurs in some patients after sexual relations with a partner infected with a different microorganism, possibly one called *Chlamydia*. In these cases a purulent (pus-like) discharge from the urethra is seen, similar to that of sexually acquired gonorrhea. Since the mechanism by which post-dysentery/ diarrhea and post-non-gonorrheal urethritis produce arthritis, conjunctivitis/iritis, and rashes is a *reaction* to a previous infection, this type of arthritis is referred to as *reactive* arthritis.

Historical recognition of reactive arthritis. Arthritis following epidemics of diarrhea or dysentery has been recognized since the time of physicians Thomas Sydenham (1624–1689) and James Lind (1716–1794), but our scientific understanding of the relationship between the two phenomena dates only to 1969.[43] People who develop arthritis after *Shigella* and *Salmonella* (and *Campylobacter* and *Yersinia*, other rod-shaped bacteria) infections of the gastrointestinal tract frequently have a gene, the histocompatibility antigen HLA-B27. Those with arthritis after one outbreak of *Shigella* infection may have diarrhea, urethritis, arthritis and conjunctivitis for up to 10 years after the inciting infection:

> It has been calculated that the likelihood of a B27-positive patient developing…[reactive arthritis] varies from 16 to 37 percent and that a B27-positive patient has a 50 times greater risk of developing arthritis after *Yersinia* infection than a person who is not B27-positive.[44]

Since persons of African descent almost never carry the B27 gene, and most of the soldiers during the Civil War were Caucasian, reactive arthritis probably comprised much of the rheumatic disease that occurred in both armies.

Reactive arthritis after sexual activity was described accurately as early as 1824, in *Lancet*, the noted British journal probably present in most medical libraries during the Civil War. All urethral discharge was called *gonorrhea* until Neisser identified the round-shaped (gonococcal) bacterium, *Neisseria gonorrhoeae*, in 1879. Thereafter post-sexual urethral discharge was referred to as gonococcal urethritis if the gonococcus was identified in the discharge and non-gonococcal urethritis if it was absent therein. The causative germ of the latter, *Chlamydia trachomatis*, was not isolated until 1957. The insightful description of a Dr. Cooper in 1824 follows, as he quotes his patient, "A gonorrhea with me is not trifle; for in a short time…you will find me with inflammation in the eyes…[and] rheumatism in the joints." Cooper gives the following account of his patient's illness: Three days after "he had a green [eye] shade on [to diminish severe light sensitivity caused by iritis, much as sunglasses would be used today], and ophthalmia [irritation] of each eye. In three days more, painful stiff knees. The rheumatism continued many weeks afterwards."[45] Of the 44 case reports of rheumatism in the war, there are six cases of probable post-dysentery/ diarrhea reactive arthritis. Three appear below:

> **Case 3**. W.W., age 32. Admitted 8–19–1862 with diarrhea of unknown duration; 2½ months later, developed fever, headache, and painful joints. By day 3 no fever; day 4 joint swelling subsiding; fever returned day 5 and continued until day 7. Swelling lessened but record does not reveal when com-

pletely gone. Acetate of ammonia begun on day 5 until day 9; colchicine given day 1 and given for 4 months. Considered "cured" after 4 months but given "light duty in the ward" until 10 months after arthritis began. Also treated with flaxseed poultices to joints, cinchona, iodide of potassium, Dover's powder (ipecac and opium),[46] sulphate of magnesia. Pain sufficient to require opium. At discharge, not returned to duty, but to Invalid Corps. Duration of symptoms: 4 months (?). *Satterlee Hospital, Philadelphia, Pa.*[47]

Comment. Case 3 received colchicine and cinchona as therapy for his arthritis. Joseph Carson in 1851 taught his medical students at the University of Pennsylvania about colchicine's "beneficial impression in gout and rheumatism."[48] Colchicine (derived from the autumn crocus) is used today to prevent and treat attacks of gout and pseudogout (types of arthritis caused by sudden release of crystals of uric acid and calcium pyrophosphate, respectively, into the joint), and plays a role in the treatment of other rheumatic diseases such as sarcoid, Behcet's Disease, Familial Mediterranean Fever, and amyloid. Quinine, obtained from cinchona bark during the Civil War, was used not only to treat malaria, but also as a bitter tonic in many types of rheumatic disease.

Case 17. W.A.E., age 22. Admitted 8–10–1862, with chronic rheumatism affecting the limbs, after diarrhea during the Peninsular campaign (late June, 1862), since which he "was much reduced in strength and flesh. The diarrhea after a time yielded to astringent and tonic treatment but the rheumatism continued;" no redness or swelling of joints, and pains more in bones than joints. Returned to duty 3–4–1863. Duration of rheumatic symptoms: 9 months. Discharged for gunshot wound right foot 4–23–1864. *Satterlee Hospital, Philadelphia, Pa.*[49]

Comment. Control of the diarrhea in Case 17 was attributed by the doctor to his treatment. This is a good example of "true, true, but unrelated," a situation in which one phenomenon, e.g. cessation of diarrhea, is observed to occur after an intervention, in this case the use of astringents and tonics, and cause and effect are therefore assumed. In fact, most diarrheas affecting soldiers at that time would have been self-limited, as the contaminated food or water-induced disease was controlled either by the body's defenses or simply "ran out of steam" on its own.

Case 40. A.T.H., age not given. Admitted 3–6–1864, with history of conjunctivitis since 11–12–1863. Both eyes inflamed and painful within a few days of each other, "feeling as if grains of sand were incommoding the [eye] ball." 5–10–1864 "Eyelids granular; vision imperfect; iris inflamed. Patient cannot read longer than fifteen minutes at a time; on a dull day he is unable to recognize an acquaintance at fifty paces; objects at a hundred paces appear double." 6–30–1864 "Cornea injected. The lids everted [turned inside out] every third day and painted with…nitrate of silver in…water." 8–7–1864 "Diarrhoea for a few days. Gave anodynes [pain reliever less potent than a narcotic] and astringents." 8–14 "Diarrhoea persisting; articular rheumatism manifested in the lumbar region and in right knee." 8–21 "Easier; some debility." 8–31 "Rheumatic ophthalmia recurring; flakes of lymph…in aqueous humor; iris hazy and sluggish; cornea clouded; vessels much injected, especially those around the upper half of the cornea." 9–16–1864 discharged from service "at which date he was suffering from intense photophobia [light sensitivity because of involvement of the iris and pupil], being unable to keep his eyes open long enough to see anything, even if the condition of the aqueous humor and cornea had permitted him to see." Duration of rheumatic symptoms: 10 mos. eyes; 7 days joints (following 7 days of diarrhea). *Kansas City Hospital, Mo.*[50]

Comment. The treatment in Case 40 consisted of silver nitrate applications to the inner eyelid. Silver nitrate is still dropped into the eyes of newborns to prevent gonococcal eye infection, which can occur during passage through the birth canal of an infected mother. This would not have been beneficial in cases of post-dysentery reactive arthritis with conjunctivitis or iritis, since the mechanism is an abnormal immune response by the host and not an infection of the eye.

Apart from case reports relating dysentery and diarrhea to arthritis, there are comments from physicians, like Surgeon W.W. Brown, 7th New Hampshire Infantry, dated 6–30–1862, which indicate familiarity with this entity and reveal that he was an astute observer:

> Most of the twenty-three cases left at Fort Jefferson, Tortugas, Fla., were rheumatism…; some of the men were quite feeble. Dysentery was often immediately followed by rheumatic disease. Many men, hitherto strangers to it, were disabled for several days, and nearly all who had any tendency from previous attacks were severely visited."[51]

These patients suffered from their arthritis, not for just days at a time, but usually for many months, as patients with reactive arthritis do today. Since the knees are often involved in this type of joint disease, a soldier would not have been able to walk or even stand up until the arthritis ran its course.

Figure 3 features the appearance of joints affected by reactive arthritis preceded, not by diarrhea or dysentery, but by sexually acquired non-gonococcal urethritis. Figure 4 illustrates another manifestation of reactive rheumatism that would have made it impossible for a soldier to march—bursitis of the heel. This condition usually persists for many months.

Examples of the genital rashes that accompany reactive arthritis are shown in Figures 5 and 6. Finally, in Figures 7 and 8 are examples of conjunctivitis that accompany reactive arthritis.

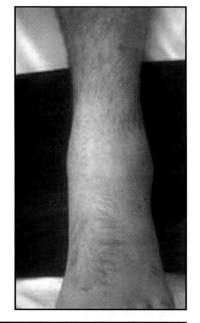
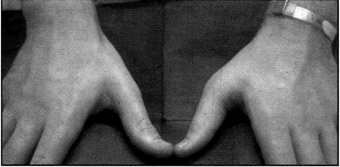

Figure 3. This 27-year-old Viet Nam veteran developed severely painful swelling in his left ankle and a swollen left thumb, two weeks after sexual contact. Non-gonorrheal urethritis preceded the arthritis by three days. Antibiotics were useless in this case of reactive arthritis, since the painful swollen joints are caused by an immune reaction to the sexually transmitted infection, and not by bacteria invading the joints. *Author's collection.*

Figure 4. Partial X-ray of the right ankle of a 29-year-old male with reactive foot pain. He has had severe right heel pain for three months. Note heel spur (arrow). Heel pain with this "moth-eaten" spur of bone is so characteristic of reactive bursitis following sexually transmitted non-gonococcal urethritis that it is called "lover's heel." X-rays were not in use until 1895. *Author's collection.*

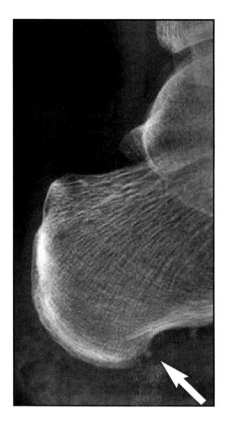

Figure 5. Mild lacy raised rash (balanitis) surrounds the opening of the urethra in the patient whose joints are shown in Figure 3. The veteran was unaware of his penile rash because it was painless and subtle. *Author's collection.*

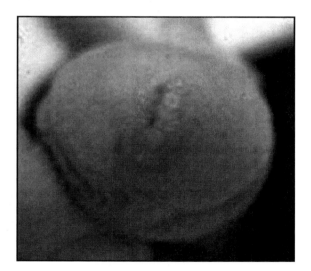

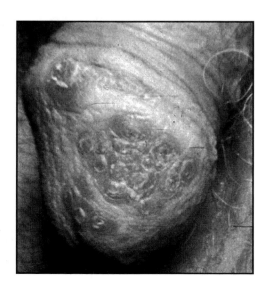

Figure 6. This balanitis would be more difficult to miss. *1972–1999 American College of Rheumatology Clinical Slide Collection. Used with permission.*

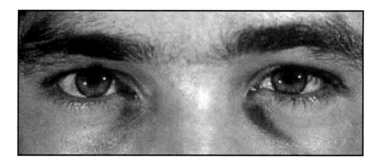

Figure 7. Conjunctivitis involving both eyes. Note dark streaks in right eye, outer aspect, caused by swelling of blood vessels. Eyelashes of both lower lids are matted together because of a pus-like discharge. The discharge does not grow bacteria, because it results from an immune reaction to the same infectious agent that is causing diarrhea/dysentery or non-gonococcal inflammation of the urethra. *1972–1999 American College of Rheumatology Clinical Slide Collection. Used with permission.*

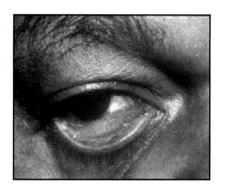

Figure 8. In this patient with post-dysentery conjunctivitis the blood vessels are clearly visible. Swelling of the vessels brings them closer to the conjunctival surface so they appear red against the white sclera. *1972–1999 American College of Rheumatology Clinical Slide Collection. Used with permission.*

3. Serious spine inflammation (ankylosing spondylitis). This type of arthritis can accompany reactive arthritis or occur by itself. It usually affects Caucasian males, if not in their adolescent years, almost always before the age of 35. The disease begins with gradual pain and stiffness in the lower back and sacroiliac joints. Unlike mechanical back pain that is relieved by bed rest, patients with ankylosing spondylitis walk around to "walk off" their pain and stiffness. They frequently suffer with an anemia, called the *anemia of chronic disease*, reflecting the generalized nature of the disease. Patients suffer also from significant fatigue and weight loss when the disease is active. If all this weren't enough, they can develop deforming arthritis of their hips, shoulders, or knees and blindness from involvement of the iris. Like its close relative, reactive arthritis, ankylosing spondylitis is associated with the HLA-B27 gene. After many years, the entire backbone, from the pelvis to the nape of the neck, may become encased in bone (fused, or ankylosed) in a severely deformed, forward-bent position. Until bioengineered therapies emerged in 1999, soldiers of all subsequent wars who developed this disease while in the service met the same fate that befell soldiers of the Civil War.

There are descriptions of this disease in Civil War troops, such as this superb one by Joseph Woodward:

> The disease begins with malaise, languor, and general indisposition to exertion. By-and-by vague pains make their appearance in various portions of the body. ... They may be located in any part of the body, but their most common seat is in the thighs and legs, and in the small of the back. The last is especially the characteristic seat of the disorder, and is more uniformly involved than any other portion of the body.
>
> The pain and soreness is at first slight, so that although the patient may occasionally come to the surgeon for treatment, he continues to do military

duty. Very often indeed he does not apply for treatment at all in this early stage, and when he first comes to sick-call inquiry shows that he has suffered from...pain for several weeks, or even longer.

As the disease progresses, the pain becomes more severe, and, if it is seated in the back or the lower extremities [legs], the patient becomes quite unfit for duty. Sometimes he is confined to his bed, but most frequently he hobbles about with the help of a stick. ... A peculiar pallid [pale], clay-like appearance of the countenance, a tendency toward emaciation, palpitation of the heart—especially after any exertion—the...pale tongue...are among the most constant symptoms.[52]

Another account by Surgeon J.M. Rice, 25th Massachusetts, New Berne, N.C., on 3-10-1863, says that "Rheumatism affecting the spinal region, hip and legs is of frequent occurrence and obstinate in its character, yielding slowly to treatment."[51]

There is one case report of a soldier who probably had ankylosing spondylitis among the 44 with rheumatism written up in the *Medical and Surgical History of the War of the Rebellion* [MSHWR].

Case 30. A.L. age 34. Admitted 4-22-1863, no duty since 1-1863, after rheumatism onset 11-1861. Right hip, thoracic spine at T-10 [thoracic, chest part of the spine].... Discharged 4-11-1864 "because of permanent contraction of the anterior abdominal and thoracic muscles following rheumatism." Duration of rheumatic symptoms: 30 months. *Satterlee Hospital, Philadelphia, Pa.*[53]

Figures 9 and 10 illustrate the typical deformities as they evolve over a quarter of a century.

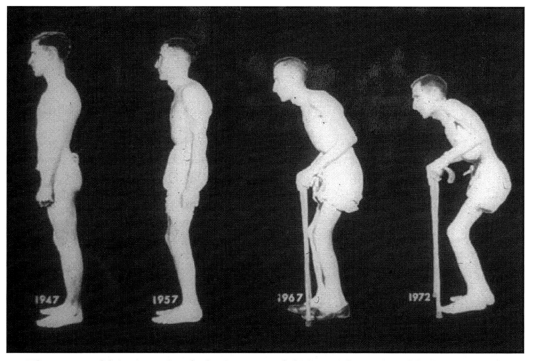

Figure 9. The natural history of ankylosing spondylitis, with inexorable formation of a "bamboo spine" in a patient. This arthritis usually affects males 17 to 35 years of age. *1972–1999 American College of Rheumatology Clinical Slide Collection. Used with permission.*

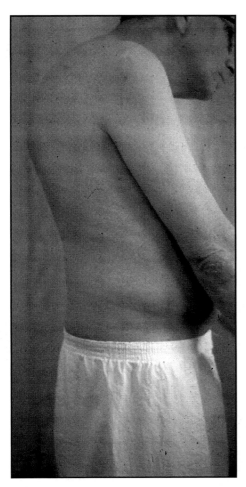 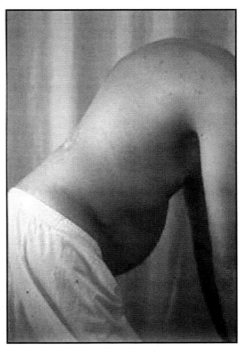

Figure 10. World War II veteran with ankylosing spondylitis, onset at 22 years of age. Left, patient is standing as straight as he can. Right, same subject, attempting to touch his toes. Note that the C-shaped curve of his lower spine looks the same whether he stands up or bends forward because it is fused (frozen) into one position. *Author's collection.*

Quite apart from this seriously deforming form of back pain many soldiers, particularly the infantrymen, would have suffered mechanical lower back pain from the punishing weight of the load he had to carry. Typically he would have had a knapsack, gun and accompanying supplies, canteen of water, blanket/bedroll, eating utensils and haversack.

4. The arthritis of scurvy (scorbutic arthritis) occurs when foods containing vitamin C are not eaten. It causes bruising of the skin, but more importantly, bleeding into joints and under the periosteum (lining around bones). Experiments conducted eighty years after the Civil War began showed the consequences of vitamin C deficiency and time of their onset:[54]

90 days:	fatigue
134 days:	corkscrew hairs, bleeding when pulled out
161 days:	bleeding around hair follicles, or petechiae ("paprika spots," the result of bleeding into the skin) over the lower legs
180 days:	petechiae over the thighs
182 days:	failure of wounds to heal
5½ months:	weight loss 27 pounds

The same study showed that the Minimum Daily Requirement of vitamin C was a measly 30 mg/day.[54]

Surgeon General of the Union Army (April 1862 to August 1863) William Hammond described his findings in soldiers and its treatment:

> Scurvy was known to the ancients, cured, as at present, by the use of fresh vegetable food. [Those with scurvy have] swollen and discolored gums, bleeding patches of...blood, first upon the legs...; hardness and [a] permanent state of contraction of the muscles; ...stiffness of the joints; ...reopening of old ulcers and cicatrices (scars)... Stiff joints [should be] rubbed with a stimulating liniment and be forcibly extended and fixed by mechanical means (splints to straighten them).[55]

The treatment of scurvy figured as a milestone in scientific medicine, having been studied in one of the earliest controlled studies ever conducted. James Lind (1716–1794) served as surgeon in the British Royal Navy from 1739 to 1748 and saw considerable scurvy. On board the *Salisbury* at sea, Lind chose twelve patients with equally severe scurvy, grouped them in twos and on May 20, 1747, administered one of six remedies to each group. The "treatments" consisted of cider, vinegar, seawater, elixir of vitriol (water and alcohol mixed with various salts of sulfuric acid), oranges and one lemon, or a mixture of nutmeg, garlic, mustard seed, balsam of Peru and gum myrrh. The two men given oranges and lemons were completely cured of their scurvy; cider resulted in some improvement also. None of the other substances had any effect on the disease.[56] Despite such an unambiguous result, standard issue of lemon juice in the British navy was delayed until 1785.[57]

5. Tuberculosis. One percent of patients infected with tuberculosis will develop infection of the spine or joints.[58] Like rheumatic fever and other conditions with chronic "rheumatism", tuberculosis made it impossible for a prospective soldier to serve in the military. John Ordronaux, in his *Manual of Instructions for Military Surgeons*, explained how to examine for Pott's disease (spinal tuberculosis):

> This affection is one of very serious consequence, in a military point of view. It reveals itself by a prominence and bulging of the spinous process (bony knob along the back of the spine), corresponding to the vertebra which is its seat.... [T]o discover the disease, the patient must be made to bend forward, while the hand is passed over the spine, to test its sensibility, and to examine critically any abnormal protuberances or depressions which may be encountered.[59]

Of the 44 case reports of arthritis, one is of tuberculosis:

> **Case 36**. G.P. age not given, U.S. Colored Troops. Admitted 12-7-1864, with "diarrhoea, cough and chronic rheumatism." By 2-8-1865 "able to walk about" despite "pain in the loins and shoulders." That evening "he had a chill with intense cardiac pain" and shortness of breath; heartbeat was 150/minute, and "dulness [sic] (heart? lung?) with a friction sound and bellows murmur." Died 2-10-1865. Autopsy: "lower lobe of each lung, the omentum (membrane passing from the stomach to other organs in the abdomen), spleen and kidneys were tuberculous; the mesenteric glands (lymph nodes in the abdomen) enlarged. There was recent pericarditis..." Duration of rheumatic symptoms: longer than 2 months (?). *L'Ouverture Hospital, Alexandria, Va.*[51]

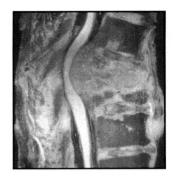

Figure 11. Side view of a post-mortem specimen affected by Pott's disease, tuberculosis of the thoracic spine. Two vertebral bodies have been destroyed. The cheesy mass filled with the causative bacterium has grown so large that it presses against the spinal cord (white vertical ribbon-like structure), causing paralysis of the legs. The over lying spine is severely deformed, assuming the shape of a right angle (gibbus) instead of the shallow C-shaped contour of the normal thoracic spine. *1972–1999 American College of Rheumatology Clinical Slide Collection. Used with permission.*

Comment. This soldier may have had "Poncet's Disease," a generalized arthritis. A more common form would have been Pott's disease of the spine or a single joint not in the spine, rather than multiple joints.

The destructive process and the resulting deformity of spinal tuberculosis are shown in Figure 11. Civil War surgeons were trained to look for this "gibbus" deformity. Prospective soldiers with no grossly visible deformity were instructed to bend forward while the examiner felt along the bony knobs (spinous processes) for a sharp protuberance. Either finding prevented military service, since the disease was so disabling.

Photographs of veterans of another war, Viet Nam, in Figures 12, 13 and 14 on facing page show tuberculosis of sites other than the spine and examples of swollen lymphatic glands characteristic of the disease, alluded to in the autopsy in Case 36 above.

The diagnosis of tuberculosis was facilitated by placing a skin test on his forearm using tuberculin. Robert Koch, who discovered the bacterium that causes the disease and proved that it did so in 1882, developed tuberculin in 1890. He hoped in vain that tuberculin would cure the disease; when it did not, Koch devised its use as a diagnostic aid. Four years after that, Wilhelm Roentgen discovered X-rays, providing further diagnostic methods for detecting this serious disease. The first effective treatment, streptomycin, did not appear until 1944. Since the tuberculosis bacterium becomes rapidly resistant to antibiotics, the disease is always treated with two or more antibiotics at a time. Drugs such as para-amino salicylic acid, isoniazid, and ethambutol were not available until 1946, 1952 and 1961, respectively.[60] Therefore, like soldiers of the Civil War, those of later wars often died of their disease.

6. Septic arthritis (pus in a joint). Septic arthritis refers to the sudden painful swelling of a joint caused by a bacterium growing within it, producing pus in the joint and a high fever in the patient. Bacteria that commonly produce this entity are staphylococci, streptococci, and others that inhabit the large intestine. The infecting bacterium is usually carried into the joint space via the bloodstream when bacteria normally confined to the skin, bowel, mouth, or teeth escape into the circulation. Less frequently, bacteria are inoculated directly into a joint from a foreign body or penetrating wound. Although tuberculosis causes pus in joints, the course is indolent rather than sudden and does not usually include high fever, as seen above. Gonorrhea is another entity causing pus in a joint, but its implications and presentations are sufficiently different that they are treated as a distinct entity.

Figure 12. Tuberculosis of the right breastbone-collarbone (sterno-clavicular, or S-C) joint in a 35-year-old Viet Nam veteran. The arrow shows his normal left S-C joint. *Author's collection.*

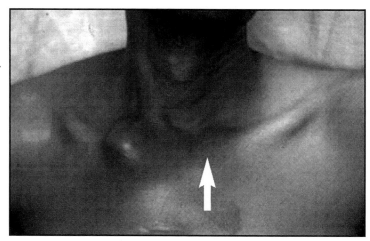

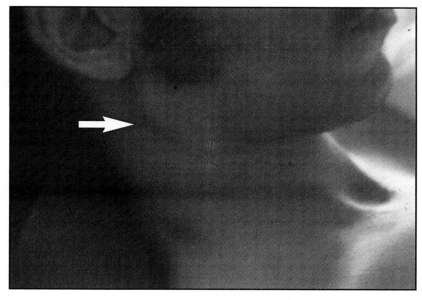

Figure 13. Swollen lymph nodes (scrofula) in a 30-year-old veteran of the Viet Nam war. He had tuberculosis of the lung, and of the right elbow—shown below. *Author's collection.*

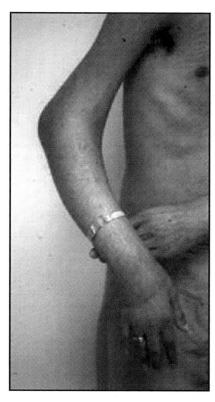

Figure 14. Right: This patient presented with a cool, very swollen but not terribly painful right elbow joint of six weeks' duration. This indolent course with swelling out of proportion to pain is very different from having a joint infected with staphylococcus ("staph"), streptococcus ("strep"), or gonococcus, which becomes swollen and unbearably painful in just a few hours. *Author's collection.*

Chapter V

In 90% of patients with septic arthritis only one joint is involved. The patient appears ill, has fever, has severe pain in the affected joint, and often has signs of an infection elsewhere. Staphylococcus is the most common cause now. During the Civil War, bacteria would have been introduced via simple skin abrasions or through wounds inflicted by missiles. Joseph J. Woodward, who received his M.D. degree from the University of Pennsylvania School of Medicine in 1853, was familiar with this devastating arthritis. He cites these particulars from a case reported in 1835:

> [In] the course of a fatal dysentery, in a man 21 years old, all the joints became successively painful and some of the seat of purulent infiltration (accumulation of pus); the right knee and left wrist were laid open by a bistoury (a long narrow knife for slitting cavities).[61]

Of the 44 cases of rheumatism recorded in the *Medical and Surgical History of the War of the Rebellion (1861–1865)*, three illustrate septic arthritis.

> **Case 7**. G.S.R., age 24. Admitted 8–29–1864 with "much fever…; his wrists and ankles were swollen, painful, tender and doughy;" morphia needed. Unchanged until 9–2 when pulse weakened, wrists became fluid-filled, many small abscesses appeared on face and chest. By 9–3 breathing and swallowing difficult, patient spit up rust colored sputum, dullness found over both lungs. On 9–4 developed erysipelas on face, pulse 130, feeble, new abscesses occurred. By 9–5 patient experienced delirium, cold clammy skin, spreading erysipelas. Expired 9–7. Autopsy: pus in both wrists, pus under the skin of an arm, signs of pneumonia both lungs, pus in spleen. Duration of symptoms: 7 days. *Hospital, Frederick, Md.*[27]

Comment. In most cases of septic arthritis only one joint is involved. This soldier suffered massive bacterial seeding into several joints, into the skin (abscesses), and into the lungs (pneumonia). Erysipelas, a dramatic red, raised streptococcal infection that spreads atop the skin, appeared late in his course, three days before his death. Even with modern antibiotics, the mortality rate in such a situation is very high.

> **Case 43**. W.P., age 42. Onset 9–1862, of right hip joint swelling "after exposure to cold and wet." Admitted 11–28–1862, with right hip pain, inability to walk without a cane. 11–1862 swelling "lanced, bringing away about four ounces of pus," and afterwards "a tablespoonful of matter…away daily." On 12–1, less swelling. Cavity was "injected with chlorinated soda in distilled water; at least four more injections until 12–15." On 12–16 "tumor (general term for swelling; here, filled with pus) enlarging, painful"; 12–22 "discharge pretty constant; high fever at night." 12–29–1862 died. Duration of rheumatic symptoms: 3 months. *West End Hospital, Cincinnati, Ohio.*[61]

Comment. The source of this man's septic hip joint is unknown. It could have been caused by an abrasion of the skin, through which bacteria entered with subsequent pressure from lying on the ground. Attribution of arthritis to "exposure" during inclement weather was common before bacteria were recognized as causes of infection in joints. Drainage of a pus-containing joint by needle aspiration or via an arthroscope remains a cornerstone of treating septic joints today.

Case 44. C.M.D. age 22. Admission date not given, but incision over right hip area was done in mid June of 1862, evacuating "about two quarts of pus...." Onset occurred after "several hours in the rain" on 4–18–1862, with "severe pain in his right hip, the whole of the gluteal region becoming swollen, tense and tender; some fever ...[accompanying] the local inflammation." By 9–1862 "abscess had healed" but pain made patient "unable to bear his weight on the limb...." He also had dullness over lower half of right chest, and rales with dullness in left lung and a [cardiac] murmur. Discharged 9–1862. Duration of rheumatic symptoms: longer than 5 months. *Hospital, Quincy, Ill.*[62]

Comment. Chest abnormalities are an ominous sign and suggest this young soldier developed pneumonia in both lungs and possibly endocarditis (cauliflower-like growths containing bacteria on one or more heart valves), almost certainly leading to his death soon after being discharged from the army.

Figure 15 demonstrates septic arthritis contracted in a different war. The elbow has been splinted in a plaster cast for comfort, but a large area remains exposed to permit needle drainage of the pus produced by bacteria that are trapped in the joint. Contact of pus with the cartilage that surfaces the bones that form the joint is very deleterious, since chemicals called enzymes are produced during the infection that can destroy cartilage within a few hours.

Figure 16 shows a sample of pus from the same patient, which has been subjected to a dye, permitting initial identification under the light microscope of the staphylococcal ("staph") bacterium responsible for his septic elbow.

Final identification and susceptibility to an antibiotic are possible in twenty-four hours when the bacterium grows on a sterile glass culture plate (Petri dish, introduced by Richard Julius Petri in 1887[63]). Robert Koch proved that one bacterium causes one infectious disease in 1878, but until Hans Christian Joachim Gram developed the stain that bears his name in 1884, distinguishing one type of round bacterium (coccus) from another was impossible. The stain causes some types, such as staphylococcus to become blue (Gram positive) and others, such as gonococcus to turn red (Gram negative) thereby distinguishing between causative bacteria. The veteran, whose purulent joint fluid is shown on the following page, experienced a full recovery. Sadly, the penicillin that cured him was not available until 80 years after the Civil War.

Mortality of septic arthritis in adults today is still high, ranging from 10% to greater than 50%.[64] Current management consists of:

- Drainage of pus from the joint by needle and syringe, using sterile technique, to remove chemicals produced during infection which destroy cartilage and bone
- Examination under a light microscope of a drop of the pus on a

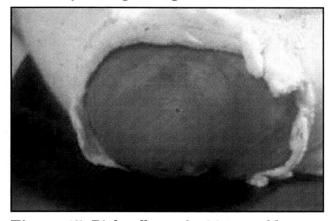

Figure 15. Right elbow of a 36-year-old previously healthy Viet Nam War veteran. In just a few hours, he experienced the sudden onset of severe pain, swelling and redness in the joint. *Author's collection.*

- glass slide stained with the Gram stain, to visualize the shape and coloration of the causative bacterium

- Removal of blood from the patient's vein for growth in the laboratory to detect bacteria that may have "seeded" (been carried into) the joint

- Administration of antibiotics by intravenous injection, based on the bacterium seen by microscopy

- Placement of pus using sterile technique onto solid gelatin-like material (culture medium) which will nourish growth of the infecting bacterium in the laboratory

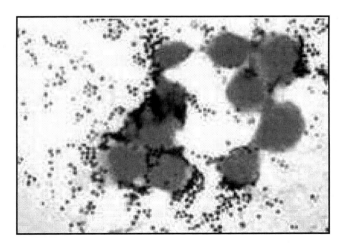

Figure 16. Distinct dark clumps of round particles ("staph") can be seen in the pus removed from the elbow in Figure 15. The large gray structures are dying cells in the joint. *Author's collection.*

- Definitive identification of the bacterium after several hours of growth ("being cultured")

- Further refinement of choice of antibiotic if the bacterium is not killed on culture by the antibiotic chosen initially

- Drainage by incision in the operating room if needle drainage cannot empty all pus from the joint

- Treatment of any accompanying infection (pneumonia, abscess, etc.)

- Institution of physical therapy to prevent contraction of a joint or other deformity arising from swelling or failure by the patient to use the joint because of pain.

Details of each step in the treatment of septic arthritis, as well as its history, appear in Appendix IV.

Narcotics for relief of pain, drainage of pus from a septic joint, removal of a foreign body which might have introduced the infection, and amputation of a limb to prevent dissemination of the infection if the affected joint were part of an arm or leg, would have been the only treatments available to the Civil War soldier with septic arthritis. Unlike soldiers with other rheumatic diseases, the natural history of which might permit them to return to duty after a variable period of convalescence, most of those unfortunate enough to contract septic arthritis died or were rendered disabled by deformity or amputation. Not until penicillin was introduced during World War II, eighty years later, would this outcome change.

7. Gonococcal ("gonorrheal") arthritis, two patterns. John Ordronaux, M.D., wrote the following in 1863:

> *Arthritis...*, when simple and recent, justifies neither rejection nor discharge [from military service] whatever may have been...its origin, whether accidental or *gonorrheal* [emphasis added], with the exception...of...the shoul-

der or hip joint, which are often serious, and demand all the attention of the surgeon. These diseases, when chronic, are...always causes for rejection, and sometimes for discharge.[65]

Gonococcal arthritis is the designation given today to arthritis that follows sexually transmitted infection with the bacterium, *Neisseria gonorrhoeae*. This differentiates this type of rheumatism from that caused by *Chlamydia*, described under *Reactive arthritis*, above. Gonococcal arthritis presents clinically in two different ways. The more common picture is sudden severely painful swelling of a single joint, often a knee or an ankle, a few days after experiencing painful discharge of pus from the urethra. The urethritis is shown in Figure 17 and the arthritis in Figure 18.

With penicillin, the infected knee pictured in Figure 18 improved rapidly. In soldiers serving in the Civil War, World War I, and World War II before penicillin became available for widespread use in early 1944, the knee joint would have been destroyed, and fatal heart infection and meningitis could have followed the gonorrhea.

The second type of arthritis resulting from the gonococcus is usually seen in men having sex with men. Because the mouth and the anus harbor the bacterium without producing major symptoms, it can grow and spread into the bloodstream. This type of infection affects many joints and may lead to meningitis or infection of the heart valves (bacterial endocarditis) if not treated promptly with antibiotics. The characteristic rash, most prominent on the hands and feet, is seen in Figure 19.

Physicians of the Civil War era, like Freeman Bumstead, clearly distinguished gonorrhea from syphilis. In addressing the treatment of gonorrhea, he states: "The idea that gonorrhoea is dependent upon the syphilitic virus and requires the use of mercurials, is without foundation."[66] This use of *virus* is not the same term used today which denotes an infectious

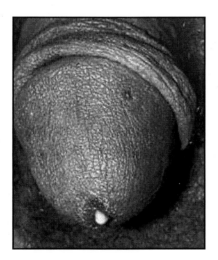

Figure 17. Typical gonorrhea, with pus draining from the urethra. A soldier with this manifestation—the typical presentation of gonococcal infection—knows he is infected and seeks medical attention promptly. Consequently, infection of a joint is usually confined to a single joint, frequently the knee. *From C. Celum, W. Stamm, Seattle STD/HIV Prevention Training Center, University of Washington. Reproduced by permission.*

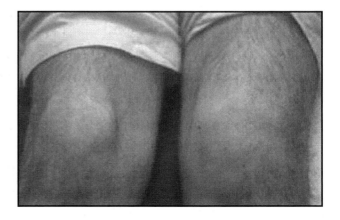

Figure 18. Painful left knee swelling in a 32-year-old Viet Nam veteran. Gonorrhea similar to that shown in Figure 17 above began three days before. *Author's collection.*

Chapter V

agent so small that it cannot be seen by a light microscope with which bacteria are seen, but must be identified using an electron microscope. Bumstead advocates that the following be done to treat gonorrhea:

> A weak solution of nitrate of silver...injected [into the urethra] until the discharge becomes thin and watery, ...before acute symptoms have set in; internally, a free purge at the outset, followed by laxatives if necessary to insure a daily evacuation from the bowels; alkaline mixtures, as solutions of the carbonates of soda or potassa, the acetate or chlorate of potassa, liquor potassae, etc., and copaiba [used as a diuretic, or stimulant]...; medication, both external and internal, ...[being] continued for ten days after all discharge has ceased; or [treatment of] acute prostatitis...at its commencement by absolute rest, cups followed by poultices to the perineum, warm baths, and laxatives or enemata...; [or opening any abscesses]...either with a knife through the rectum, or with the point of a catheter through the urethra.[67]

None of these interventions would have prevented the disabling arthritis arising from gonococcal infection not treated promptly with an antibiotic, since it results from spread through the bloodstream before the joint pain and swelling even appear. Bumstead's entire treatise on the treatment of gonorrhea, as well as its prevention, appears in Appendix V.

8. The arthritis of syphilis. The behavior of syphilis after it is acquired by sexual contact is complex. A few weeks after sexual exposure, a *primary stage* occurs. The hallmark of this period is a genital ulcer called a *chancre*, seen in Figure 20. The chancre is associated with swollen lymph glands in the groin.

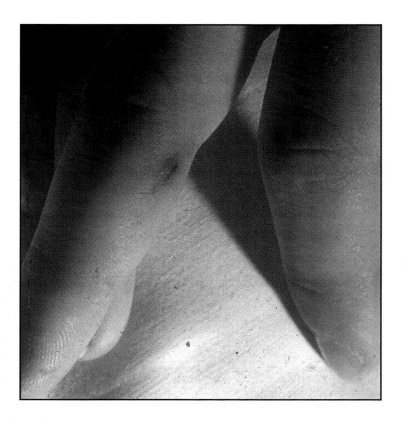

Figure 19. Blood blister on a finger, seen typically in gonococcal arthritis acquired by men having sex with men. The veteran of the Viet Nam War whose rash is shown above had unprotected anal intercourse four days before the rash appeared on his fingers and toes, accompanied by severe arthritis and tendonitis in his wrists, knees, shoulders and ankles. *Author's collection.*

The chancre is highly infectious to the owner (and any sexual partner). Unlike chancres in other sexually transmitted diseases, the edges of the syphilitic chancre are firm to the touch, much like the consistency of the end of the human nose. If primary syphilis is not treated with systemic antibiotics, secondary syphilis results.

Physicians of the Civil War period were aware of, and characterized well, the first stage of this infectious disease. Bumstead describes primary syphilis:

> There is always an interval between the appearance of the chancre and of the general manifestations of syphilis. This period of incubation of general symptoms...is fixed within certain bounds, like the incubation of other infectious diseases. Its average duration is six weeks....[68]

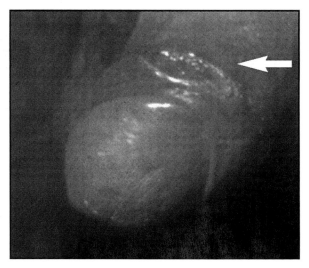

Figure 20. The chancre (ulcer) of syphilis is painless. If a soldier did not examine himself, he might not realize it was present. *Photograph courtesy of H.M. Leavitt, M.D. and N.M. Matus, M.D.*

What they did not, nor could not, realize was that the germ that causes the disease, a spirochete, spreads very quickly to the bloodstream. If not treated with antibiotics, secondary syphilis results, since the infection spreads internally beyond the chancre within hours or days of infection, even before the chancre appears. It is during this stage of secondary syphilis that arthritis may appear, along with rashes in the mouth and on the skin, malaise (sense of not feeling well), fever and swollen lymph glands throughout the body. Dr. Bumstead gives an equally insightful picture of secondary syphilis:

> Early general symptoms...consist of an eruption of blotches...upon the skin, ...*mucous patches...of the mouth*...general malaise, headache, and *fleeting pains* in various parts of the body, [more particularly in the neighborhood *of the joints*,]....[69]

The "patches" inside the mouth are illustrated in Figure 21 on the following page.

Secondary syphilis has been associated with joint pain and swelling in several reported series. Ankles and small joints of the feet were the most common in a report in 1916.[70] Swelling and pain in one joint, or both knees predominated in another, published in 1932.[71] In 6 of 144 cases of secondary syphilis reported in 1976, prominent symptoms included aching pains in bones in the back, arms and legs.[72] In a study of seven patients with tendonitis of the wrists and ankles, and arthritis affecting knees, ankles, fingers and the sternoclavicular (collarbone and breastbone) junction, structures suggestive of degenerating spirochetes were seen with an electron microscope.[73] Another in 1989 recorded an 18-year-old male who developed pain and swelling in the right ankle for two days, and subsequently in both knees. Unlike others with joint pain during secondary syphilis, this young man had

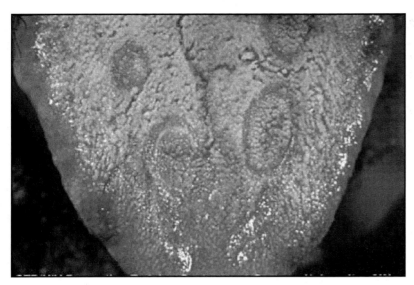

Figure 21. The "mucous patches" of secondary syphilis are seen here on the tongue. *Reproduced by permission of the Seattle STD/HIV Prevention Training Center, University of Washington.*

no fever and no rash. On careful questioning, however, he recalled a chancre four months before his joint pain began, which he ignored.[74]

Not known until 1903 was the next stage of the infection, a period of no complaints by the patient and no abnormal findings on physical examination, denoted *latent syphilis*. This stage is only detectable by blood tests, the earliest of which was the Wassermann test. Many soldiers would have been serving in the Civil War as their latent phase evolved. They and their surgeons would reasonably have interpreted the disappearance of syphilitic symptoms as a "cure," and attributed the cure to whatever treatment had been rendered. The final stage of infection, *tertiary syphilis*, requires several years to develop[75] and involves the aorta, brain and spinal cord. Therefore, unless they were infected before the Civil War, the troops would not have manifested symptoms of tertiary syphilis.

Definitive treatment was not available until Ehrlich introduced Arsphenamine, or Salvarsan, an arsenic derivative, in 1909.[76] The use of mercury to treat syphilis, as well as four other diseases during the war will be covered in Chapter IX, *Mercury after Venus*, and Chapter VIII, *Mercury without Venus*.

9. Rheumatoid arthritis (RA). This disease involves multiple joints and may lead to severe deformity and disability after just a few years. Commonly there is a symmetric pattern of the swollen, painful, tender joints, i.e., both knees, both wrists, small joints of both hands and both feet. The patient with RA experiences marked stiffness each morning on arising and may not "loosen up" until noon; he is also plagued with fatigue every day.

Studies of Bannatyne in 1896 were among the earliest to describe RA and distinguish it from other deforming types of arthritis, such as gout.[77] Its cause, an immune reaction gone awry in which the patient's own joints are attacked, damaged and destroyed, was recognized only 50 years ago.[78] Gold salts and chemotherapy such as methotrexate became the mainstay of therapy for the latter half of the twentieth century. A more detailed understanding of the events leading to the destruction characteristic of RA finally led to bioengineered immune therapy in 1999.[78]

Four cases that might be rheumatoid arthritis in Civil War soldiers appear below.

Case 5. A.M. age 52. Admitted 4-5-1864, "suffering from rheumatism while at home on furlough. Knees and wrists swollen and painful; swelling extending from knees down the legs." By 4-9 needed laudanum [a narcotic]. By 4-12 swelling "much reduced; slight pain in ...[front of chest] but no change in sounds." 4-24 given laudanum "for external use." 4-26 swelling and pain "much diminished." May 15 swelling in arms returned. June 1 arms and hands very swollen, until June 15 when "somewhat reduced." By July 28 regaining "use of arms slowly; wrist-joints stiff. Transferred to 16th and Filbert Streets...." Diagnosis "acute rheumatism." November 29th transferred to Haddington, diagnosis "chronic rheumatism." Feb. 18, 1865 discharged "because of chronic rheumatism causing distortion and deformity of joints of fingers of both hands and left knee-joint." Treated with Dover's powder, colchicum, laudanum, potassium iodide, tincture of aconite, iron, quinine, joints packed in lint soaked in sodium bicarbonate, wet cupping "drawing about an ounce and a half of blood," pressure bandages warm bath, external tincture of iodine. Duration of symptoms: 10 months. *South Street Hospital, Philadelphia, Pa.*[62]

Comment. Syringes, as seen in Figure 22, were used in the Civil War, sometimes to administer narcotics under the skin. In this case opium, part of Dover's powder, was given by mouth. Another component of Dover's powder, ipecac, was used to induce sweating in cases with inflammation (swelling, warmth, redness, pain) or fever, to remove injurious substances from the blood. Cupping removed such substances by drawing blood into a blister formed by suction of the glass "cup." Quinine was given not only for malaria, but also for other causes of fever. Aconite (wolfsbane, or monkshood) was employed as a sedative if given by mouth; as an irritant if applied to the skin. Colchicum (colchicine) remains a useful treatment today for several rheumatic diseases.

Case 25. J.W. #25, age not given. Admitted 1-20-1864, after several months of rheumatism in knees, ankles, neck and shoulders. "He was stout and well-built, yet worthless as a soldier." 8-31-1864 able to do light ward duty; transferred to another hospital 10-12-1864; returned to duty 10-28-1864. Duration of rheumatic symptoms: longer than 12 months (?). *Kansas City Hospital, Mo.*[79]

Comment. Note that this soldier's arthritis rendered him unable to fight for 9 months. His return to duty may reflect the tendency of rheumatoid arthritis to subside spontaneously for varying periods of time in most patients. This characteristic waxing and waning of pain, swelling and stiffness in rheumatoid arthritis makes it difficult to evaluate treatment even today. The question often arises: Did the patient improve because of therapy, or because the disease quieted down ("went into remission") on its own?

Case 27. J. McM. age 32. Admitted 4-27-1863, chronic rheumatism with pallor, anemia, "feeble and unable to walk on account of the swelling of his joints." Slowly improved but unable to walk; transferred to Invalid Corps 11-25-1863. Duration of rheumatic symptoms: longer than 7 months (?). *Hospital, Quincy, Ill.*[79]

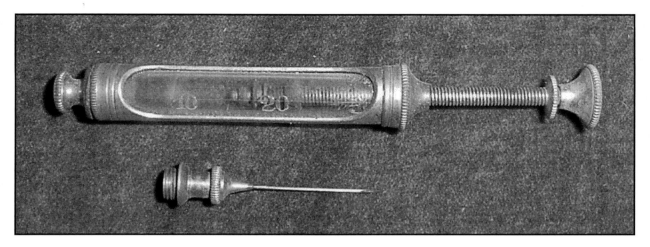

Figure 22. Syringes of the Civil War period were made of glass. *Courtesy of the National Museum of Civil War Medicine.*

Comment. Pallor, or paleness, is caused by a lack of red cells in the bloodstream resulting in less pink coloration of the skin. The term anemia for this condition is still used today. This anemia has the same cause as that seen in *Serious arthritis of the spine, ankylosing spondylitis*, discussed earlier in this chapter—ongoing activity of certain chronic diseases. The anemia contributes to the lassitude of these patients (less oxygen-carrying capacity of the red blood cells), and disappears only when the arthritis becomes inactive (in remission) because of treatment or by virtue of the natural history of the disease.

> **Case 28**. V.S. age not given. Onset rheumatism about 1855 for several months. Served 18 consecutive mos. in the field until 10–1862, when second attack occurred, affecting knee and elbow joints. Admitted one year later, 10-24-1863, when "much thickening of the tissues about the joints, with exquisite pain on motion." Best return of function was 1-25-1864, when walked with cane. "There was no heart disease. He was discharged from service" 4-9-1864. Duration of rheumatic symptoms: longer than 18 months. *Central Park Hospital, New York City.*[53]

Comment. This man almost certainly had his first attack of RA seven years before this episode, followed by spontaneous remission before deformity of his joints occurred. Hence he would not have been rejected for service by the army's examining surgeon. Had deformities been present, he would have been pronounced unfit for military service. The notation, "no heart disease" is the reporting surgeon's way of saying that this arthritis was not caused by rheumatic fever. Without heart failure, listening for murmurs with a stethoscope would have enabled that conclusion. Figure 23 shows that the degree of swelling in joints affected by RA may be great. Obviously a soldier with this would not be able to march nor kneel to fight. He would have difficulty even changing position in bed or going to the toilet. Deformities following long-standing RA can be seen in Figure 24.

10. Malaria. Malarial rheumatism is expressed as fever, muscular aching, backache and joint pain.[80] Although there are no case reports of this entity, it is clear that it was recog-

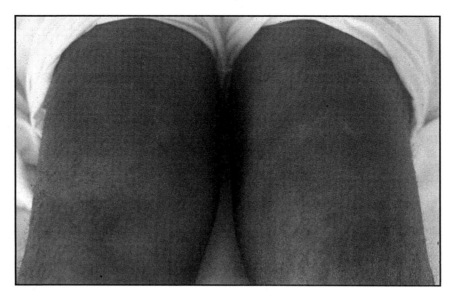

Figure 23. Significant swelling of both knees in a Viet Nam War veteran with, at age 29, the onset of pain, swelling and stiffness in both knees, stiffness in both wrists, the small joints of the hands and feet, the ankles, and the shoulders. Despite injections of gold salts and an oral antimalarial drug (hydroxychloroquine), he was unable to care for himself or to work. *Author's collection.*

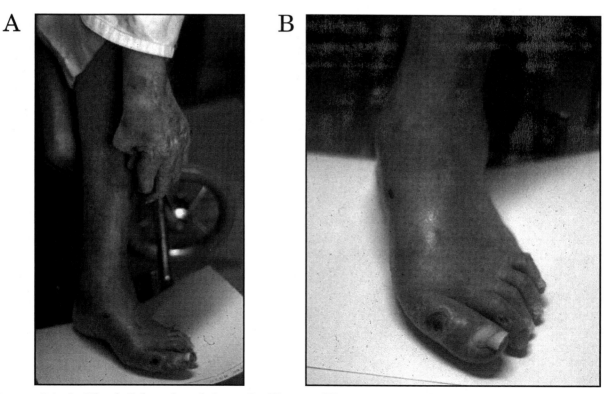

Figure 24. A. The left hand and foot of a Korean War veteran with rheumatoid arthritis. After ten years of the disease, he was unable to dress or bathe himself, and could move about only in his wheelchair. B. Detail of his ankle and foot deformities. His opposite foot appears the same, except that he had no ulcers on the right foot. *Author's collection.*

nized as a significant problem among the troops. Surgeon A.H. Lanphier, 106th Illinois Infantry, wrote from Jackson, Tennessee, on New Year's Eve of 1862:

> Resident physicians tell me they have more rheumatism and intermittent fever than all other diseases together. I suppose that the low swampy surface of the country will account for this fact. It is customary here to give large doses of quinine in acute rheumatism, and the practice is by no means unsuccessful.[81]

Lanphier's comments illustrate how medical information was acquired during the war by surgeons stationed in areas unfamiliar to them: they asked the local doctors. Word-of-mouth experience, not controlled studies of a large series of patients with a disease, provided guidance. Lanphier's allusion to the low swampy location shows clearly that he accepted the prevailing "mal (bad) air" theory of disease, that many diseases were caused by poisonous fumes arising from decaying vegetation and swampy areas. The true cause of malaria, a parasite carried by a specific type of mosquito, would not be discovered until three years before the nineteenth century ended. The mosquito vector is shown in Figure 25.

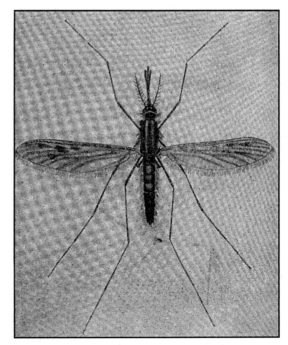

Figure 25. The female anopheles mosquito, indicted in 1897 as the vector of malaria by Dr. Ronald Ross. *Source: Mason CF. A Complete Handbook for the Sanitary Troops of the U.S. Army and Navy and National Guard and Naval Militia, 4th ed. New York: William Wood and Company; 1918: 357.*

There is ample evidence that mosquitoes abounded in warm weather and annoyed the soldiers during the Civil War. At the Andersonville Prison Hospital, Sumter County, Georgia, in 1864 the problem is described thus: "Myriads of mosquitoes…infested the tents, and many of the patients were so stung by these pestiferous insects that they appeared as if they were suffering from a slight attack of measles."[82] U.S. Sanitary Commission Document #69 lists as supplies during and immediately after the Battle of Gettysburg 648 pieces of mosquito netting @ $810.00. The price of the netting was the same as that for 4,000 dozen eggs.[83]

Although quinine was used extensively in the treatment of malaria, it was also used frequently in rheumatic diseases not associated with malaria. Assistant Surgeon, C.S. Wood, 66th New York, wrote on September 30, 1862:

> Rheumatism was quite prevalent at Yorktown from cold and exposure to wet. The ordinary anti-rheumatic remedies had very little effect; colchicum and guaiacum were tried in vain. Taking it for granted that this was due to a malarial complication, I used a cathartic, followed by a grain of opium and five of quinia, every four or six hours, with the happiest effect.[84]

The concept that rheumatism was caused by exposure to cold wet weather is echoed in a Confederate account. "A major in the Jeff Davis Legion seeks reassignment to an Alabama regiment so that he will not have to winter in Virginia. Over a year of campaigning and sleeping on wet ground has caused him great suffering from rheumatism."[85] The role of exposure as a promoter of rheumatic diseases persisted well into the twentieth century. Dr. Ralph Pemberton (1877–1949), called the "Father of Rheumatology" by many, attributed the majority of the rheumatic diseases occurring in veterans of World War I to such exposure.

11. Gout. Gout is one of the best understood of the more than 100 types of rheumatic disease. Caused by a very sharp and irritating crystal of uric acid, it is responsible for some of the most painful arthritis that humans experience. One rare form appears in early life and has nothing to do with obesity. The more common form occurs in later life and is seen frequently in the obese. Ordronaux, as usual, is on target with his observations:

> Gout is extremely rare in youth, being generally found only in old age. It is also…infrequent…among soldiers and non-commissioned officers, whatever may be their age. It would, if present, constitute a disqualification for the military service.[86]

In order to distinguish it from other rheumatic diseases, gout was denoted by a separate diagnostic number in *The Sickness and Mortality Reports* in *The Medical and Surgical History of the War of the Rebellion (1861–1865)*. In the Union Army there were 137 conditions enumerated from the first day of the war until July 1, 1862, when the number increased to a final of 152 diagnoses. Each disease and type of injury was identified with a unique number; acute rheumatism was #36; chronic rheumatism, #37. Gout was not a common cause of arthritis, judging from the quarterly reports to the Surgeon General of the U.S. Army, as shown below.

Table IV. Arthritis Attributed to Gout[87-92]

White Troops:			
Cases the first year of the war	104		
Cases, second year	158		
Cases, third year	103		
Cases, fourth year	102		
First year after the war	28	Total	495
U.S. Colored Troops:			
Cases, 1863–64	0		
Cases, 1864–65	4		
Cases, 1865–66	3	Total	7

Figure 26 shows a Korean War veteran with gout in several joints of his right foot. This severe episode of gouty arthritis was controlled with cortisone, non-steroidal anti-inflammatory drugs (NSAIDs) and colchicine. Civil War surgeons used colchicine to treat several types of arthritis, but cortisone was unknown until 1949. The first NSAID, phenylbutazone, was not available until 1950.[93] That same year it became possible to prevent gout, and not merely treat an attack after it occurred, with the development of probenecid.[93] Such an episode of gouty arthritis would have been very disabling in battle. The usual attack of gout lasts for two weeks. During this period the soldier would have found any footsteps toward or away from his bed unbearable, since vibration brings on excruciating pain in the involved joints. There would have been no possibility of his leaving his bed to go to the toilet. Even blowing air on his foot or toes would have made the pain unbearable. There being widespread hunger at various periods of the war on both sides, gout associated with obesity would have been mercifully rare.

There is a problem accepting gout as a diagnosis in soldiers of the Civil War. It was a decade after the war ended until gout could be distinguished from other chronic deforming types of arthritis. Alfred Baring Garrod made this possible in 1876, when he used a polarized light microscope to visualize uric acid crystals, which are unique to gouty arthritis.[94] Furthermore, the gold standard for diagnosing gout—removal of fluid from a painfully swollen joint with a needle, and identification of uric acid crystals with a *compensated polarized microscope* to distinguish the crystals of gout from other crystals that can cause arthritis—was not established until 1962, a century after the Civil War.[95]

12. Mumps. Arthritis occurs during infection with mumps in 0.44 percent of patients and does so more commonly in men.[96] Gordon and Lauter describe this rheumatic disease:

> The arthritis begins from day 1 to 15 days after the onset of the parotitis (salivary glands that swell during invasion by the mumps virus), with multiple large and small joints affected. Effusions (fluid build-up in the joint) are infrequent. Symptoms subside within 2 weeks, although arthritis may persist for up to 3 months.[97]

There were 48,128 cases of mumps in white troops[91] and 12,186 in the U.S. Colored Troops[92] recorded during the war. Assuming that 0.44% developed arthritis, the Union Army would have had out of commission for up to three months 211 white troops and 53 U.S. Colored Troops (USCT), as the arthritis ran its course and subsided spontaneously. Mumps therefore accounted for even fewer cases of arthritis than gout.

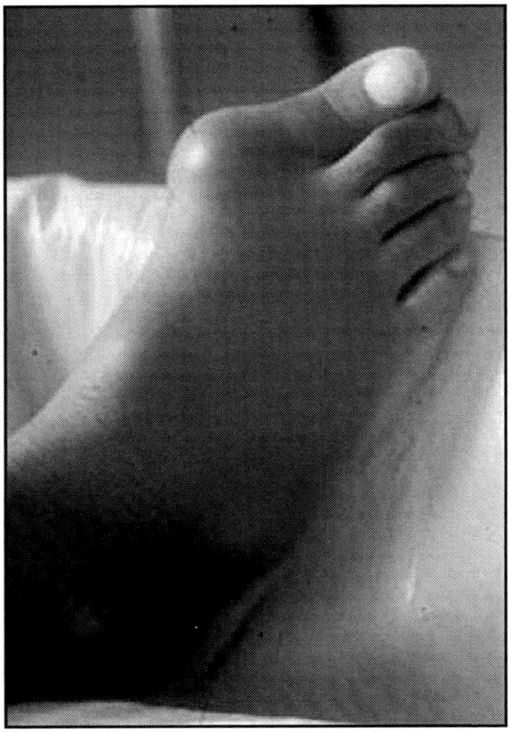

Figure 26. Gout has caused marked swelling not only in the big toe joint, commonly affected by gout (podagra) in this veteran of the Korean War, but also in his ankle and mid-foot joints. *Author's collection.*

Consequences of rheumatic diseases are shown in Tables V through X below.

Table V. Outcome of the 44 Cases of Rheumatism Reported by the Union Army[15]

Acute	Patients
Returned to duty	3
Invalid corps	1
Disability discharge	1
Death	8
Chronic	
Returned to duty	11
Invalid Corps	3
Disability discharge	10
Leave of absence	1
Death	6

Table VI. Outcome of Cases of Rheumatism Listed in the *Sickness and Mortality Reports*[98,99]

475 of 254,738	(0.19 %) Died (White)
235 of 32,125	(0.73 %) Died (USCT)

Table VII. Mortality from Rheumatism in General Hospitals in two Regions[100–107]

Ending 1862	Atlantic	1	soldier
	Central	19	
Ending 1863	Atlantic	35	
	Central	50	
Ending 1864	Atlantic	8	
	Central	66	
Ending 1865	Atlantic	147	
	Central	51	
USCT: No data given			

Table VIII. Discharge on Surgeon's Certificate of Disability of those with Rheumatic Diseases[108-109]

11,779 of 254,738	(4.6 %)	disabled (White)
874 of 32,125	(2.7 %)	disabled (USCT)

Table IX. Reasons for Discharge with Disability in U.S. White Troops, Total for the War[110]

1.	Gunshot wounds	33,458
2.	Consumption (tuberculosis)	20,403
3.	Diarrhea	16,185
4.	Debility	14,500
5.	Rheumatism	11,779
6.	Heart disease	10,636
7.	Hernia	9,002

Table X. Reasons for Discharge with Disability in U.S. Colored Troops, Total for the War[111]

1.	Rheumatism	874
2.	Gunshot wounds	751
3.	Consumption	592
4.	Debility	540
5.	Hernia	358
6.	Old age	478
7.	Amputations	327

Summary. There were considerable numbers of soldiers in the Civil War who experienced extreme pain, immobility, and even death from rheumatic diseases. The compulsive record keeping and case reporting required by the Union Army allow a glimpse into the lives of those with rheumatism. The natural history and course of several rheumatic diseases that affect young men during crowded unsanitary conditions are understood today, and they don't paint a "pretty picture." Once acquired, conditions such as rheumatic fever, or reactive arthritis, or ankylosing spondylitis, lasted several weeks and tended to return again and again, because the patient's immune system began the disease and then perpetuated it. The soldier's only means of relief would have been narcotics. Often he would have been utterly dependent on his fellow soldiers or nurses to attend to basic latrine needs, feeding, bathing and dressing. If his arthritis was not immune-based, and due solely to an infectious disease, the patient often died. Clearly rheumatic diseases took a great toll in terms of the suffering of the soldiers who experienced them and of compromising battle readiness of armies on both sides during the Civil War.

Chapter V References

1. Steiner PE. *Disease in the Civil War*. Springfield, IL: Charles C. Thomas; 1968: 7–8

2. *Ibid.*, 53–54

3. Denney RE. *Civil War Medicine: Care & Comfort of the Wounded*. New York: Sterling Publishing Co., Inc.; 1995: 41–42

4. Steiner PE. *Disease in the Civil War*, Springfield, IL: Charles C. Thomas; 1968: 111

5. *Ibid.*, 174

6. Freemon FR. *Microbes and Minie Balls: An Annotated Bibliography of Civil War Medicine*. Cranbury, NJ: Associated University Presses, Inc.; 1993: 143–144

7. *Ibid.*, 165

8. *Ibid.*, 169

9. *Medical and Surgical History of the War of the Rebellion (1861–1865)*, Medical Vol., Part 1, Vol. 1. Washington, D.C.: U.S. Government Printing Office; 1870: 146–151, 296–301, 637. Hereafter *MSHWR (1861–1865)*

10. *Ibid.*, 684–689, 710

11. *Ibid.*, 296–301, 637

12. *Ibid.*, 684–689, 710

13. *Ibid.*, 646

14. *Ibid.*, 716

15. *MSHWR (1861–1865)*, Medical History, Part 3, Vol. 1: 829–844

16. Cheadle WB. Harveian lectures on the various manifestations of the rheumatic state as exemplified in childhood and early life. *Lancet*. 1889; I: 821–827, 871–877, 921–926

17. Jones TD. Diagnosis of Rheumatic Fever. *JAMA*. 1944; 126: 481–484

18. Special Writing Group of the Committee on Rheumatic Fever...of the American Heart Association. Guidelines for the diagnosis of rheumatic fever, Jones criteria, 1992 update. *JAMA*. 1992; 268: 2069–2073

19. Krause RM. Streptococcal Diseases. In: Wyngaarden JB and Smith LH, Jr., eds. *Cecil Textbook of Medicine*, 18th ed. Philadelphia: W.B. Saunders Co.; 1988; 1574–1577

20. Kaplan EL. Rheumatic Fever. In: *Harrison's Principles of Internal Medicine*, ed. Fauci AS, 15th ed., New York: McGraw–Hill; 1998: 1340–1343

21. Bisno AL. Rheumatic Fever. In: Wyngaarden JB and Smith LH, Jr., eds. *Cecil Textbook of Medicine*, 18th ed. Philadelphia: W.B. Saunders Co.; 1988; 1528

22. Morton LT and Moore RJ. Einthoven W. In: *A Chronology of Medicine and Related Sciences*. Brookfield, VT: Ashgate; 1997: 467

23. Sydenham T. Chorea. In: Pechey J, ed. *The Whole Works of that excellent Physician, Dr. Thomas Sydenham*, 7th ed. London: M. Wellington; 1717: 417–418

24. *Medical and Surgical History of the Civil War*. Wilmington, NC: Broadfoot Publishing; Vol. 1. 1990: 646. Hereafter *MSHCW*

25. *MSHWR (1861–1865)* Part 3, Vol. 1: 829–844

26. *Ibid.*, 829

27. *Ibid.*, 831

28. Ordronaux J. *Manual of Instructions for Military Surgeons*. NY: D. Van Nostrand; 1863: 19–20

29. Hoeprich PD, Flynn NM. Chemoprophylaxis of Infectious Diseases. In: Hoeprich PD, Jordan MC, Ronald AR, ed. *Infectious Diseases*, 5th ed. Philadelphia: J.B. Lippincott Co.; 1994: 312–313

30. *MSHWR (1861–1865)* Part 3, Vol. 1: 832

31. Ordronaux J. *Manual of Instructions for Military Surgeons*. NY: D. Van Nostrand; 1863: 152

32. *MSHWR (1861–1865)*, Medical History, Part 3, Vol. 1. 1888: 831–832

33. *Ibid.*, 840

34. *Ibid.*, 837

35. *Ibid.*, 839

36. Heggie AD. Prevention of Streptococcal Pharyngitis and Acute Rheumatic Fever in Navy and Marine Corps Recruits. *Navy Medicine*. 1998; 79: 26–28

37. James L, McFarland RB. An epidemic of pharyngitis due to a non-hemolytic group A streptococcus at Lowry Air Force Base. *N Engl J Med*. 1971; 284: 750–752

38. CDC. Acute Rheumatic Fever at a Navy Training Center—San Diego, CA. *Morbidity and Mortality Weekly Report*. 1988; 37: 101–104

39. Olmstead FL. U.S.S.C. Report #40; 1861: 61

40. *MSHWR (1861–1865)* Part 3, Vol. 1. 1888: 745–749

41. *MSHWR (1861–1865)* Medical Volume, Part 1, Vol. 1. 1875: 646–648

42. *Ibid.*, 711–712

43. Ahvonen P, Sievers K, Aho, K. Arthritis associated with *Yersinia enterocolitica* Infection. *Acta Rheum Scand.* 1969; 15: 231–253

44. Smith JW. Infectious arthritis. In Mandell GL, Douglas RG, Jr., Bennett, JE, eds. *Principles and Practice of Infectious Diseases*, 3rd ed. New York: Churchill Livingstone; 1990: 912

45. Cooper A. Gonorrheal Rheumatism, *Lancet*; 1824: 301–302

46. Dorwart BB. *Carson's Materia Medica: An Annotation*. Bala Cynwyd, PA: WVD Press; 2003: 62

47. *MSHWR (1861–1865)*, Medical Vol., Part 3, Vol. 1. 1888: 830

48. Dorwart BB. *Carson's Materia Medica: An Annotation*. Bala Cynwyd, PA: WVD Press; 2003: 59

49. *MSHWR (1861–1865)*, Medical History, Part 3, Vol. 1. 1888: 837–838

50. *Ibid.*, 841–842

51. *Ibid.*, 840

52. Woodward JJ. *Outlines of the chief camp diseases of the United States Armies*. Philadelphia: J.B. Lippincott & Co.; 1863: 319–320

53. *MSHWR (1861–1865)*, Medical History, Part 3, Vol. 1. 1888: 839

54. Crandon JH et al. Experimental Human Scurvy. *N Engl J Med* 1940; 223: 353–369

55. Hammond W A. Scurvy, in *Hammond's Military Medical and Surgical Essays*, Philadelphia: J.B. Lippincott and Co.; 1864: 175–204

56. Stewart CP, Guthrie D, ed. *Lind's Treatise on Scurvy. Reprint of the first edition of James Lind of 1753.* Edinburgh: Edinburgh University Press; 1953: 145–148

57. Morton LT and Moore RJ. In: *A Chronology of Medicine and Related Sciences*. Brookfield, VT: Ashgate; 1997: 110–111

58. Evanchick CC, Davis DE, Harrington TM. Tuberculosis of Peripheral Joints: An Often Missed Diagnosis. *J Rheumatol.* 1986; 13: 187–189

59. Ordronaux J. *Manual of Instructions for Military Surgeons*. New York: D. Van Nostrand; 1863: 152

60. Morton LT, Moore RJ. *A Chronology of Medicine and Related Sciences*. Brookfield, VT: Ashgate; 1997: 763

61. *MSHWR (1861–1865)*, Medical History, Part 2, Vol. 1. 1879: 408

62. *MSHWR (1861–1865)*, Medical History, Part 3, Vol. 1. 1888: 843

63. Morton LT, Moore R J. *A Chronology of Medicine and Related Sciences*. Brookfield, VT: Ashgate; 1997: 391

64. Ho G, Jr. Septic Arthritis Update. *Bulletin on the Rheumatic Diseases*. 2002; 51: 1–4

65. Ordronaux J. *Manual of Instructions for Military Surgeons*. New York: D. Van Nostrand; 1863: 191

66. Bumstead, FJ. Venereal Diseases, in *Military Medical and Surgical Essays prepared for the USSC*, ed. Hammond, WA; Philadelphia: J.B. Lippincott and Co.; 1864: 532

67. *Ibid.*, 533–535

68. *Ibid.*, 546

69. *Ibid.*, 547

70. Wile U, Senear F. A study of the involvement of the bone and joints in early syphilis. *Am J Med Sci.* 1916; 152: 689–693

71. Kling D. Syphilitic arthritis with effusion. *Am J Med Sci.* 1932; 183: 538–548

Chapter V

72. Waugh MA. Bony symptoms in secondary syphilis. *Brit J Vener Dis.* 1976; 52: 204–205

73. Reginato A, Schumacher HR, Jimenez S, Maurer K. Synovitis in secondary syphilis. *Arthritis Rheum.* 1979; 22: 170–176

74. Kazlow PG, Beyer B, Brandeis G. Polyarthritis as the initial symptom of secondary syphilis: case report and review. *Mount Sinai Journal of Medicine.* 1989; 56: 65–67

75. Tramont EC. Chapter 213, *Treponema pallidum* (syphilis) in *Principles and Practice of Infectious Diseases*, ed. Mandell GL, 3RD ed. New York: Churchill Livingstone; 1990: 1794–1802

76. Morton LT, Moore RJ. *A chronology of medicine and related sciences.* Brookfield, VT: Ashgate; 1997: 755

77. Bannatyne GA. *Rheumatoid arthritis: its pathology, morbid anatomy, and treatment.* Bristol: John Wright; 1896

78. Rose HM et al. Differential agglutination of normal and sensitized sheep erythrocytes by sera of patients with rheumatoid arthritis. *Proc Soc Exp Biol Med.* 1948; 68: 1–6

79. *MSHWR (1861–1865)*, Medical History, Part 3, Vol. 1. 1888: 838

80. Kean BH, Reilly PC. Malaria—the mime. *Am J Med.* 1976; 61: 159–164

81. Lanphier AH. *MSHWR (1861–1865)*, Medical History, Part 3, Vol. 1. 1888: 840

82. *MSHCW* Vol. V; 1990: 42

83. USSC Document #69. New York: William C. Bryant and Co.; 1863: 60

84. *MSHWR (1861–1865)*, Medical History, Part 3, Vol. 1. 1888: 841

85. Sutherland D E. *Seasons of War: The Ordeal of a Confederate Community 1861–1865.* Baton Rouge, LA: Louisiana State University Press; 1995: 196

86. Ordronaux J. *Manual of Instructions for Military Surgeons*, NY: D. Van Nostrand; 1863: 194

87. *MSHWR (1861–1865)*, Medical History, Part 1, Vol. 1. 1870: 147

88. *Ibid.*, 297

89. *Ibid.*, 453

90. *Ibid.*, 605

91. *Ibid.*, 631

92. *Ibid.*, 710

93. Smyth CJ, Freyberg RH, McEwen C. *History of Rheumatology.* Atlanta, GA: Arthritis Foundation; 1985: 125

94. Garrod, AB. *A Treatise on Gout and Rheumatic Gout (Rheumatoid Arthritis).* London: Longmans, Green; 1876

95. McCarty DJ. Phagocytosis of urate crystals in gouty synovial fluid. *Amer. J. Med. Sci.* 1962; 243: 288–295

96. Smith, JW and Sanford JP. Viral arthritis. *Ann Intern Med.* 1967; 67: 651–659

97. Gordon SC, Lauter CB. Mumps arthritis: a review of the literature. *Rev Infect Dis.* 1984; 6: 338–344

98. *MSHWR*, Medical, Part 1, Vol. 1. 1870: 637

99. *Ibid.*, 710

100. *MSHCW*, Vol. 1; 1990: 61

101. *Ibid.*, 115

102. *Ibid.,* 199

103. *Ibid.,* 265

104. *Ibid.,* 349

105. *Ibid.,* 421

106. *Ibid.,* 605

107. *Ibid.,* 573

108. *MSHWR*, Medical Vol., Part 1, Vol. 1. 1870: 646

109. *Ibid.,* 716

110. *MSHWR* Medical Volume, Part 1, Vol. 1. 1875: 646–648

111. *Ibid.,* 716–718

Chapter VI.

Bronchitis and Catarrh

This chapter, and the one following, address upper respiratory infections and abscesses because they were among the four most common diagnoses reported in the *Sickness and Mortality Reports* of the Union Army, and as such impaired the ability of troops to march and to fight. Benjamin Franklin's observation about the transmission of the common cold was prescient. "I have long been satisfied from observations, that...people often catch cold from one another when shut up together in close rooms, coaches, etc., and when sitting near and conversing so as to breathe in each other's transpiration...."[1]

The common cold was also called catarrh by Civil War surgeons. Dunglison, in his 800 page medical dictionary of 1846, defines catarrh as "inflammation of the mucous membrane of the air-passages" and a cold as a:

> Superficial inflammation [irritation] of the mucous follicles of the trachea and bronchi. It is commonly an affection of but little consequence, but apt to relapse and become *chronic*. It is characterized by cough, thirst, lassitude, fever, watery eyes, with increased secretion of mucus from the air-passages. The antiphlogistic [agents believed to counteract irritation, such as those inducing vomiting and emptying the bowels] regimen and time usually remove it. Sometimes, the inflammation of the bronchial tubes is so great as to prove fatal.[2]

In the *Sickness and Mortality Reports* of the *Medical and Surgical History of the War of the Rebellion (1861–1865)*, there is no listing of the common cold, only catarrh. There were 83,665 cases of catarrh in all theaters between July 1, 1861 and June 30, 1862, making this diagnosis the third most common of that year.[3] As expected, colds varied widely month to month, peaking during the winter months, as shown in Table I.

The common cold, caused by a *virus*, usually lasts a week, with a "runny," stuffy nose, mild headache, sneezing and a mildly sore throat.[4] However, it can be complicated by a *bacterial* infection of the throat, airways and lungs. Because there is so much swelling of the lining inside the nose, the sinuses and Eustachian tubes (connecting the throat with the middle ear) can become blocked. The obstructed secretions then can become infected with bacteria, resulting in severe sinusitis and middle ear infections (otitis media). Without antibiotics, these secondary infections frequently would have been fatal.

Although the electron microscope, which permits visualization of viruses, was invented in 1932,[5] the first common cold virus was not discovered until 1956.[6] Colds are spread by inhaling the air exhaled by an infected person. The virus travels from person to person on droplets that are sneezed into the air. This is why colds increase in the winter months when people are in close quarters and ventilation is limited. Experiments in volunteers showed that cold weather per se, humidity, dampness, and sharp changes in temperature have no effect on the development of a cold:

Table I. Frequency of the Common Cold by Month the First Year of the War[3]

Month	Number of Cases
July	800
August	1,422
September	2,673
October	5,125
November	9,350
December	13,152
January	15,242
February	11,544
March	9,669
April	7,884
May	3,858
June	2,946

> Under natural conditions, transmission of...[viruses that cause the cold] may proceed from an infected to susceptible persons by transfer of virus via the hand, fingers, or an intermediary surface. Self-inoculation of the eyes or nose with virus on the finger may result in...the common cold [also].[6]

With rare or no regular hand washing practiced by most troops (and their surgeons), it is easy to imagine how common the common cold was during the war.

After the first year of the war, *catarrh* is no longer listed as a diagnosis, replaced by *acute bronchitis*. Dunglison (1846) defines bronchitis thus:

> Inflammation of the lining membrane of the bronchial tubes. This is always more or less present in cases of pulmonary catarrh; and is accompanied by cough, mucous expectoration, ...and...uneasiness in breathing. The *acute* form is accompanied with all the signs of internal inflammation, and requires the employment of antiphlogistics followed by repulsives. [The *chronic* form has an expectoration] which is generally mucous, although, at times muco-purulent [mucus mixed with pus].[7]

From July 1, 1862, to June 30, 1863, there were reported in the *Sickness and Mortality Reports* 60,792 cases of acute bronchitis, the fourth most common cause of illness that year in all theaters in the war.[8] Distribution by month of these cases is shown in Table II, again with a concentration highest in the winter months.

Chapter VI

Table II. Frequency of Colds/Acute Bronchitis by Month the Second Year of the War[8]

Month	Number of Cases
July	3,697
August	2,493
September	3,230
October	3,010
November	6,080
December	8,244
January	7,892
February	7,550
March	8,221
April	5,680
May	2,873
June	1,822

Most soldiers with acute (lasting less than a week) bronchitis would have recovered uneventfully from this disease, also caused by any of several viruses. As with some colds, they could develop a secondary infection—with a bacterium. Antibacterial agents able to cure the secondary infections, such as sulfa, would not be available until 1935 or, in the case of penicillin, until 1943.

Chapter VI References

1. Bayne-Jones S. *The evolution of preventive medicine in the U.S. Army, 1607–1939.* Washington, DC: U.S. Government Printing Office; 1968: 12

2. Dunglison R. *A Dictionary of Medical Science*, 6th ed. Philadelphia: Lea and Blanchard; 1846: 143–144

3. *Medical and Surgical History of the War of the Rebellion (1861–65).* Washington, DC: Government Printing Office, 1888, Medical Vol. & Appendix, Part 1, Vol. 1. 1875: 146–151. Hereafter *MSHWR (1861–1865)*

4. Morton LT, Moore RJ. *A Chronology of Medicine and Related Sciences.* Brookfield, VT: Ashgate; 1997: 719

5. Liu C. Chap. 20, The Common Cold, in *Infectious Diseases*, 2nd ed. Hoeprich PD, ed. Hagerstown, MD: Harper and Row; 1977: 221

6. *Ibid.*, 223

7. Dunglison R. *A Dictionary of Medical Science*, 6th ed. Philadelphia: Lea and Blanchard; 1846: 114

8. *MSHWR (1861–65),* Medical Vol. & Appendix, Part 1, Vol. 1. 1875: 296–301

Chapter VII.
Abscesses, Carbuncles and Boils

The current definition of an abscess is unchanged since Dunglison's in 1846: "Abscess. A collection of pus in a cavity, the result of a morbid process."[1] Today an abscess is defined as a collection of pus that is buried in tissues or organs or in some other confined space, and is accompanied by fever. A **boil** is a collection of pus in the skin with a hard central core. It is usually the result of infection by bacteria called *staphylococci* ("staph") that live normally on the skin and descend below the surface by growing along a hair follicle. A carbuncle is a collection of pus in a cluster of boils under the skin; it also is caused largely by staph. All three are painful.

Although many types of bacteria can be the infecting agent, staph is still the most common. Abscesses in the liver, spleen and lungs in Civil War soldiers would probably have been caused by *Endamoeba histolytica*. This parasite produces dysentery, which was prevalent during the war, and spreads beyond the intestine to cause abscesses in the three sites just mentioned. Boils usually drain spontaneously, but the deeper collections may not. The primary treatment of those that do not is drainage of the cavity by incising the affected area and packing the drainage site with a wick or a tube to insure that it does not close and re-trap pus. Depending on the location of the infection and the general health of the patient, antibiotics may also be prescribed. Obviously, in the 1860s, drainage and packing the cavity would have been the only options. It is remarkable therefore that there were only 180 deaths reported in the *Sickness and Mortality Reports* for the entire war in white soldiers and only 21 in the U. S. Colored Troops (U.S.C.T.) who had abscesses.[2] Numbers of cases affected by abscesses, carbuncles or boils appear in the table below.

Table I. Cases of Abscesses, Carbuncles or Boils in all Years of the War[3,4]

	White Troops	U.S.C.T
Abscesses	47,246	2,376
Carbuncles	7,560	240
Boils	78,2033	4,967

Several case reports follow, illustrating the variety of sites in which abscesses developed, the detailed records kept by the surgeons, how abscesses were treated, and the disability and mortality associated with them. Like most other case reports, these were not included in the statistics reported above, since the soldiers being reported individually were cared for in a hospital; the *Sickness and Mortality Reports* excluded hospitalized patients.

Chapter VII

Case 326. —Private William Koppen, company C, 7th New York volunteers; age 20; admitted June 5, 1865. Chronic diarrhoea. This man was excessively emaciated.... Treatment: Tonics and nourishing food. June 27th: Cod-liver oil in porter. July 1st: Severe diarrhea set in. The former remedies were then discontinued, and two grains of quinine directed thrice daily, with tincture of the chloride of iron every four hours; also milk and lime-water.... Subsequently quarter of a grain of nitrate of silver and half a grain of opium every four hours. At times the patient complained of excessive pain in the upper third of the left thigh, but could move the hip-joint on the affected side without any pain or inconvenience. July 11th: An abscess was detected in the anterior [front] portion of the left thigh.... July 15th: Assistant Surgeon William F. Norris, U.S.A., opened the abscess, evacuating a quantity of thin fetid pus. ... [Given] citrate of iron and quinia, four grains, three times daily; an ounce of sherry wine every three hours. In the evening there was high fever and profuse perspiration. July 16th: The discharge still continues; the fever and sweating have increased. July 21st: ...[Treatment]. Aromatic sulphuric acid, five drops, every three hours. July 22d: The diarrhoea is worse. July 26th: Had eight stools in the last twenty-four hours, accompanied by dysenteric symptoms. July 28th: Is losing strength; countenance sharp; profuse perspiration. July 29th: Ten stools. August 1st: Delirious. Died, August 3d, at 3:30 A.M. Autopsy ten hours after death: Body excessively emaciated. The abscess was found to extend to the...capsule of the left hip-joint. ... The lungs were healthy. The liver fatty. The spleen enlarged and softened. The kidneys normal. Peyer's patches [dense collections of infection-fighting cells that form oblong bumps on the inner lining of the small intestine] were very visible. The rectum was ulcerated, the ulcerations varying from the size of a pea to that of a large almond. The mucous membrane [the inner lining of the bowel] was thickened. —Acting Assistant Surgeon Carlos Carvallo.[5]

Comment. Dysentery after months of diarrhea resulted in "excessive emaciation" and malnutrition, reducing the body's ability to resist and survive infections that might develop. Replacement of fluid and chemicals lost in the dysenteric stools, and administration of nutrients and calories by intravenous solutions (total parenteral nutrition) was not possible until the mid-twentieth century. The earliest antibiotics that would have been effective in such cases were developed in 1935 (sulfa) and 1943 (penicillin). The high fevers and profuse perspiration in this case probably represent release of bacteria from the abscess into the bloodstream, rather than toxic effects from the abscess alone.

Surgeon Carlos Carvallo, who authored the case report above, was a member of the largest group of physicians who cared for soldiers of the war, *Acting* or *Contract,* surgeons. Except during very large battles, such as Antietam and Gettysburg, these surgeons did not serve in the field. They were hired by the army to work in general hospitals.

Case 1260. —Private W. Raper, Co. G, 5th North Carolina, was wounded at Williamsburg, May 5, 1862. On May 9th, he reached Hygeia Hospital. Surgeon R.B. Bontecou reported: "Admitted with amputation of the right leg and a gunshot wound of the right arm, the ball entering at the outer border of the biceps...and emerging behind its inner border. The leg stump...was attacked with erysipelas [then this meant either a spreading red skin infection caused by streptococcus or a deeper infection of the skin called cellulitis; now the term applies only to the former]. He was removed to a separate room in a distant portion of the building. Recovering from this, he was returned to one of the surgical wards in the early part of June, and soon complained of an abscess occupying the anterior [front] of the right shoulder. There was little pain except on motion of the arm, but the swelling was large when my attention was called to it, and although the...[skin was not] discolored [red]..., fluctuation [wavelike sensation felt on touching a fluid-filled cavity] so apparent and the wall so thin, I opened it, and a very large amount of pus, eight ounces, escaped. Three days after this, the assistant surgeon on duty enlarged the opening, and pus flowed again freely....Death ensued...June 14, 1862, ...from exhaustion, and the *post-mortem* revealed an ulceration of the brachial artery at the situation of the bullet wound... communicating with the abscess above by a sinus along the edge of the biceps. The whole [shoulder] joint was disorganized and denuded of its cartilage; the scapula [shoulder blade] seemed to float in an inner abscess.... This was likewise the case with the left scapula and joint, and the hip joints, each, were distended with pus.[6]

Comment. This example shows how severe abscesses can develop from a missile passing through a limb, how they spread via the bloodstream to several joints, and how they usually eventuate in the death of the patient. Had Private Raper survived, he would never have walked again because of destruction of his hip joints (septic arthritis); nor would he be able to care for personal hygiene, feed himself or dress himself, with destruction of both shoulders. Note that this soldier with highly contagious erysipelas was isolated from other patients on admission to the hospital. It is remarkable, without antibiotics, that he did not expire from *this* infection.

The next patient, against the odds, survived his abscess, after being in the hospital for three months. He was unable to return to duty, however.

Case 310. —Corporal S.A. Holden, Co. D, 1st Maine Cavalry, aged 19 years, received, at Upperville, Virginia, June 21, 1863, a stab by a sabre, which...[penetrated] the liver. He was taken to a neighboring field hospital in charge of Assistant Surgeon R.A. Dodson, 1st Maryland Cavalry. There was not much bleeding, but great...distension, which subsided on the tenth day, and was followed by an abscess of the liver. This was incised...[from the front of the abdomen], on July 13th, and a profusion of pus was evacuated. The patient was supported by a sustaining regimen, and, on August 2d, was sufficiently convalescent to bear transportation to the 3d division hospital at Alexandria. The wound had healed, but he was very weak. He improved rapidly, and was returned to duty on October 7, 1863; but, being unfit for active service, he was sent to Armory Square Hospital on March 20, 1864. A...hernia had protruded at the site of the cicatrix [scar].[7]

The outcome of Private Miller's liver abscess, chronicled below, was death three weeks after being wounded:

Case 456. —Private S. Miller, Co. I, 24th Missouri, aged 18 years, was wounded at Bayon De Glaize, May 18, 1864. A conoidal [minié] ball penetrated the upper surface of the right lobe of the liver and the under surface of the right lobe of the liver and the under surface of the right lobe of the lung. He

Chapter VII

was treated in the hospital of the 3d division, Sixteenth Corps, until June 2d, when he was transferred, on the hospital boat N.W. Thomas, to St. Louis, and admitted to the hospital at Jefferson Barracks. Stimulants and anodynes [pain relieving drugs less potent than an anesthetic or a narcotic] were there administered. Pyaemia [bloodstream infection leading to multiple abscesses] was developed, and death resulted June 8, 1864. At the necropsy, a large abscess was found in the right lobe of the liver, containing about four ounces of pus. Two thirds of the lower lobe of the right lung were solidified [pneumonia was present]. The case is reported by Surgeon John F. Randolph, U.S.A.[8]

Not all bullets were removed from soldiers, but those lodged in the abdominal wall almost always were. Dr. George A. Otis explains why:

> It is especially important to extract…[foreign bodies] from the abdominal walls; for they rarely become encysted there; the action of the muscles and disposition of the sheath [enclosing the muscles] facilitating…movement [of the ball]; the liability to abscess-formation in propinquity to the peritoneum presenting a constant source of danger while they remain. The course of balls, making a long track, was indicated by a red or reddish-blue line, when they passed beneath the skin or first layer of muscles. It was sometimes necessary to make an incision for the evacuation of pus…at the middle of the track; but it was considered injudicious to lay open the canal, the seton wounds healing sooner, as a general rule, than the furrowed wounds.[9]

A "seton wound" was made by passing a thread or a wire through the skin into an abscess, creating a passage to drain the pus. The seton sometimes was left in place for the rest of the soldier's life, depending on the location of the abscess. Dr. Otis, who was in Walter Brice's medical school class of 1851, at the University of Pennsylvania, was an eminent surgeon during the war. He was chosen to write the surgical volumes of the *Medical and Surgical History of the War of the Rebellion (1861–1865)*. He died before completing all of the three volumes.

Chapter VII References

1. Dunglison R. *A Dictionary of Medical Science*, 6th ed. Philadelphia: Lea and Blanchard; 1846: 13

2. *Medical and Surgical History of the War of the Rebellion (1861–65)*. Washington, DC: Government Printing Office, 1888, Medical Vol. & Appendix, Part 1, Vol. 1. 1875: 641, 712

3. *Ibid.*, 641

4. *Ibid.*, 710

5. *Medical and Surgical History of the Civil War*. Wilmington, NC: Broadfoot Publishing; Vol. III; 1990: 155. Hereafter *MSHCW*

6. *MSHCW* Vol. IX; 1991: 444

7. *Ibid.*, 129

8. *Ibid.*, 137

9. *Ibid.*, 12

Chapter VIII.
Mercury without Venus: Mercurials in the Treatment of Non-Venereal Diseases

Alfred Stillé informs the readers of his two-volume text, *Therapeutics and Materia Medica*, published in 1860, that the Greek name for mercury (quicksilver) is *hydrargyrum*, because at "ordinary temperatures" it is a "shining liquid."[1] Accordingly, the scientific symbol for this metal is Hg (hydr, water; argyros, silver).

There are over 400 documented cases in *The Medical and Surgical History of the War of the Rebellion (1861–1865),* in which mercury was prescribed for ill soldiers. Apart from using mercury as a cathartic, the surgeons caring for these men did not administer mercury in a random way, but for a highly-selected group of diseases. They obeyed the standard of care for their time that was based on published guidelines and a detailed rationale for this treatment. The five conditions for which mercury was used were dysentery or diarrhea, typhoid fever, malaria, pneumonia, and syphilis. This chapter details the use of mercury in the first four conditions. The role of the metal in syphilis will be covered in the chapter that follows.

Dysentery or diarrhea. Although *The Medical and Surgical History of the Civil War* records more than 1.7 million cases of dysentery and diarrhea in its Field Reports of U.S. White Troops and U.S. Colored Troops,[2] there are only 859 case reports of soldiers with diarrhea or dysentery in this source. Sixty-two of these 859 men received mercury.[3] A typical case of dysentery (bloody diarrhea with painful spasms of the anal sphincter, resulting in an urgent desire to empty the bowels, but without producing feces) is that of Private Nales:

> **Case 279**. —Private Thomas Nales, company A, 71st Pennsylvania volunteers; age 26; admitted March 5, 1863. This man was much emaciated; pulse 60 and feeble; tongue furred, white in the centre, edges red, papillae raised. He had from ten to fifteen bloody purulent looking stools [pus in the bowel movements] daily; there was severe pain in the lower abdomen, and tenderness on pressure, with anorexia [lack of appetite] and much thirst. Treatment: Blue mass [composed of mercury, confection of roses, and powdered liquorice root], opium, solution of…iron, sulphate of quinia [quinine], milk-punch, &c. Died, April 5th. *Autopsy*: The body was much emaciated; the abdomen flat and sunken. There were pleuritic adhesions [lining around the lungs was scarred] on both sides. The heart was normal. The liver pale; the gall-bladder much distended. The spleen was four and a half inches long by two and three-quarters wide. The kidneys normal; the bladder distended with urine. The mucous membrane of the stomach and small intestine was much congested. The colon was much thickened, and there were patches in its lower portion. The rectum was ulcerated throughout.[4]

A second case was not treated with mercury. An illustration of the soldier's colon accompanies this report. The surgeon who performed the autopsy prepared the large intestine and sent it to the Army Medical Museum in Washington, D.C., an institution begun at the outset of the

Chapter VIII

Civil War to document the illnesses and injuries occurring during the war. The collection was divided into medical and surgical sections. Specimens from soldiers who died of an illness, in contrast to those obtained after a surgical procedure, became part of the medical section.

Case 893. Army Medical Museum #703, Medical Section. "Private W. Brooks, company H, 2d United States colored troops; enlisted March 11, 1865. From this time till December 31, 1865, he appears on the muster-rolls of his company as present for duty, except during September and October, when he was on detached service. With the exception of these two months he served in Florida, and was under treatment by the regimental surgeon for constipation, and in July and August for jaundice. About the middle of December he was taken sick with dysentery, and in January was sent north for treatment. He was admitted to Harewood hospital, Washington, D. C., January 12, 1866, having been sick four weeks. He had the usual symptoms of acute dysentery, and died January 20th. Was not much emaciated at the time of death. The treatment consisted of astringents, opiates and supporting measures. *Autopsy*: The small intestine appeared to be quite normal. The colon was thickened and ulcerated in many places throughout. The rectum as in the specimen. The condition of the other organs is not recorded.
—Surgeon R. B. Bontecou, U. S. V.[5]

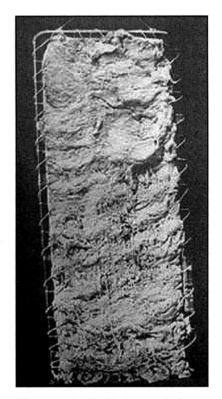

The specimen from Private Brooks can be seen in Figure 1. The picture is a heliotype, "made by printing directly from a gelatin film exposed under a negative and hardened with chrome alum."[6] This particular heliotype was made for the Army Medical Museum by James R. Osgood & Co., in Boston.

This case is especially important because the description of ulceration and pseudomembrane is identical to the modern description of bacillary (caused by the *Shigella* bacillus) dysentery, as illustrated by Dr. Frank Netter in 1962.[7]

Typhoid fever. This is a serious disease caused by a different rod-shaped bacterium, a kind of *Salmonella*, but <u>not</u> the one that causes food poisoning. Cardinal features of the disease are several weeks to months of sustained fever in the range of 105°, headache, mental confusion, red flushing of the face, nosebleed, bronchitis, an enlarged spleen, abdominal pain, constipation or diarrhea (but not dysentery), and a characteristic rash on the abdomen and chest called "rose spots."

Of the 79,462 cases of typhoid fever listed in *The Medical and Surgical History of the Civil War* (*MSHCW*),[8] only 119 detailed reports appear there. Of these, 44 men

Figure 1. Heliotype of the rectum of Case 893, showing ulcers and a "pseudomembrane." The latter is a false membrane consisting of large sections of the inner lining of the bowel that pull away during this serious infection. *The Medical and Surgical History of the War of the Rebellion (1861–1865)*.

received mercury as part of their treatment.[9] The following account is of Private George Barber who survived the ordeal and returned to duty 27 days after his disease began. Barber was one of 51 soldiers diagnosed with typhoid fever and cared for in the Seminary Hospital, Georgetown, D. C., during the autumn and winter of 1861, under the supervision of Surgeon Joseph R. Smith, U.S.A. Cases were received from the Army of the Potomac. This series reported a death rate of 19.6 percent.

>**Case 9**. —*Deafness; dizziness, but mental faculties clear; diarrhea; rose-colored spots on the 10th and 12th days, fading on 14th, when convalescence followed; to duty on 27th day.* —Private George N. Barber, Co. G, 14th N. Y.; age 18; was admitted Sept. 20, 1861, having been taken sick a week before with weakness, pains in the head, back and bowels, and epistaxis [nosebleed]. Diagnosis—typhoid fever. On admission the pulse was 114, the skin hot and moist, the face flushed, the tongue gray in the centre and red at the tip and edges; there was diarrhea, with irritability of the stomach and much tenderness in the right iliac region [right lower part of the abdomen]; the patient was sometimes affected with dizziness, but his mind was clear. Blue-pill [mercury, liquorice root, confection of roses] was given. On the 21st he had five stools with persisting tenderness with gurgling, anorexia [loss of appetite], a slight cough, epistaxis and deafness; his face was flushed, skin hot and moist, tongue red at tip, whitish-gray at base. On the 22d the epistaxis recurred; the tongue was dark-red at the tip, brown at the base, and its papillae [taste buds] were prominent; the skin was warm and dry and presented one or two rose-colored spots; one stool was passed…; pulse 76. Quinine in eight-grain doses was given three times daily, with morphia [an opiate] at night. The eruption faded next day, but appeared again on the 24th. The tongue began to clean on the 22d and the skin softened on the same day, after which, although the bowels continued relaxed and tender for a few days…, there was a steady improvement, and the patient was returned to duty October 9.[10]

In the case above mercury was administered only once. A second patient from the same series was given multiple courses of mercury.

>**Case 15**. —*Mental dulness* [sic]*; delirium; eruption* [rash]*; diarrhoeal affection not prominent as a symptom; skin moist; date of onset not defined.* — Private Frederick P. Seclor, Co. A, 9th Pa.; age 24; had suffered from fever and ague [aching] in June 1861; but since then had done his duty uninterruptedly until September 19, when he was admitted as a case of typhoid fever. In the evening the patient was weak and had headache; the bowels were quiet, but there was some tenderness in the right iliac region [lower abdomen] and intestinal gurgling; face flushed; eyes bright; breath offensive; pulse 88; skin hot and moist; head cool and sweating; tongue grayish-yellow in the centre, red and clean at the edges. Ten grains of calomel [mercurous chloride] and jalap [dried root which acts as a cathartic] were given. Next day, with a continuance of the symptoms stated, the patient became dull and stupid and had…tinnitus [ringing in the ears]. On the night of the 21st there was delirium, and the characteristic eruption appeared on the 22d, on which day also he had two stools with…tenderness [in the abdomen]…. Turpentine emulsion and wine were given. Next

Chapter VIII

night he was again delirious, and on the 23d dull, the skin unaltered save by the fading of the eruption [rose spots] from the chest and abdomen, the bowels quiet, …but free from tenderness, and the tongue cleaning. Dover's powder [potassium sulfate, ipecac, and opium] was given in small doses, with stimulants. An enema was administered on the 24th, with two grains of blue-pill and one of quinine every three hours. By the 26th the eruption had disappeared, but the patient continued dull; the skin was moist, the tongue cleaning. The bowels were moved once on this day and on the 27th, and some tenderness…remained; but after this the tongue became clean, the appetite good and the bowels natural. The patient was returned to duty October 20.[11]

Malaria. Another disease with high fever that plagued the troops was malaria. Unlike the fever in typhoid fever (constant), fever in malaria is intermittent. If fever occurs every three days, it is called quartan; if every two days it is tertian; if daily, quotidian. Because the parasite (plasmodium) that causes malaria ruptures the red blood cells in which it grows and reproduces, the patient becomes anemic and pale. Liver involvement may cause the patient's skin to become yellow (jaundiced; icteric). Surgeon Joseph J. Woodward gives an insightful description of the disease in his 1864 book, *Outline of the chief camp diseases of the United States Armies*. "The complexion is…icteroid in hue, and a peculiar anemic pallor, with the evidences of hepatic disorder, permits at once the recognition of…chronic malarial poisoning."[12]

Civil War surgeons connected the disease with hot weather, marshes, and standing water. They believed it to be caused by vapors (mal air) arising from decaying vegetation. Not until Sir Ronald Ross' work in 1897 was the correct mechanism of disease causation known: a parasite living in a specific mosquito (*Anopheles*) that was inserted via a mosquito bite into a human from another human already infected with malaria. The mosquito that carries the parasite is illustrated in Figure 25, in Chapter V.

Although the *MSHCW* records 982,611 cases of malaria (defined as Intermittent Fever: Quotidian, Tertian or Quartan),[13] there are detailed records of only 102 soldiers with malaria. Of these, 21 were prescribed mercury by their surgeons in the U.S. Army.[14] Two of these case reports appear below.

Case 4. *A quartan with slow recovery after several relapses*, Private James Wright, Co. F, 21st Ill. Vols.; age 21; was admitted September 25, 1863, having a chill every third day. His skin was sallow, tongue coated and bowels loose. Strychnia, blue-pill [mercury rubbed with confection of roses, beaten with powdered liquorice root][15] and capsicum [derived from peppers] were prescribed. He improved slowly, suffering several relapses; ultimately Fowler's solution [arsenic and potassium; used as an alterative, intended to alter the natural history of a disease without obvious loss of a bodily substance] proved effectual and the patient was returned to duty February 14, 1864. —*General Hospital, Quincy, Ill*.[16]

There is no evidence that arsenic kills the malarial parasite. Note that the surgeon assumed, because the soldier improved after treatment with arsenic, the arsenic was the reason for the improvement. Before controlled studies were used to test medical treatments, such assumptions commonly established medical practices. Quinine, an effective treatment, was used widely during the Civil War to treat malaria. This case is unusual in that Private Wright was not given quinine.

Case 19. *"Tertian becoming quotidian...."* "Lieutenant H. M. Rideout, 10th U. S. Art'y [Artillery], was admitted November 3, 1863. He had been attacked ten days before with a severe chill, followed by fever and headache; two days after this he had a second chill with fever and some delirium. The fever was accompanied with much pain in the back, anorexia, gastric [stomach] irritation, prostration and constipation. The chill recurred daily during the next three days. After the fifth chill there had been only imperfect remissions of the fever. The patient had been on duty for eight months in the low swampy lands of Louisiana. On admission his pulse was 120 and skin hot, dry and pallid [pale]. Ten grains of blue pill were given, and quinine and capsicum ordered every three hours. Under this treatment the fever abated and there was no recurrence of the chills. On November 9 there was slight fever, the pulse 96..., but this condition lasted only a few hours. He was returned to duty on the 30th. —*Hospital, Natchez, Miss.*[17]

Treatment of malaria with cinchona bark, the source of quinine, was practiced in Peru as long ago as 1630.[18]

Pneumonia. Figure 2 shows the appearance of a lung affected by pneumonia. Although pneumonia can be caused by several types of bacteria and by viruses, the patients so infected all have a cough, fever, sputum production, variable chest pain and difficulty breathing. *The MSHCW* records 77,335 cases of pneumonia (listed as *inflammation of lungs*).[19] Of these, the clinical course of 118 soldiers is reported.[20] Mercury was prescribed for 14 of these. A typical case was reported by Surgeon Peck on New Year's Eve, 1862:

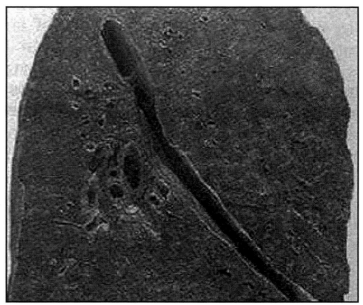

Figure 2. The lower portion of the lung is less dense because it is not infected, and the normal lung cells are filled with air. The upper part appears much more solid because pus, not air, fills the cells. *Photograph courtesy of R. Ochs, M.D.*

Case 3. —There was but one case of pneumonia during the past quarter,–a violent case in a dissipated subject. The patient stated that the day before he had a chill which was followed by fever and cough, with much pain in the side, so severe that he could scarcely breathe and did not sleep any during the night. He had violent cough with the characteristic rusty sputa [material brought up by coughing had the color of rust]; severe pain in the left side; great dyspnoea

Chapter VIII

[difficulty breathing]; high fever; intense headache; pulse full, strong and frequent; skin hot and dry; face livid and anxious; respiration hurried; bowels constipated and urine scanty. 1st day: Gave four compound cathartic pills [colocynth (dried bitter apple), jalap, gum-resin, and mercurous chloride] and applied a blister over the seat of pain [an irritating substance placed on the skin caused a blister filled with fluid; the fluid thus produced was presumed to contain the noxious agent that caused the chest pain, drawing it out of the body]. 2d: Bowels well opened; the blister relieved the severe pain in the side; other symptoms unaltered. Gave brandy, eight ounces, morning, noon and night, with good nourishment. 3d: Very restless and sleepless during the night; symptoms unchanged. Gave twenty grains of sulphate of quinia [quinine], with half a grain of tartar emetic [antimony potassium tartrate, to induce vomiting], morning and evening; continued brandy and beef-tea. 4th: All the symptoms much improved; fever subsiding; pulse soft; skin moist; breathing easier; sputa mingled with less blood; secretion of urine copious. Diminished the quinia and tartar emetic by one-half; continued brandy and beef-tea. From this day complete convalescence was established and the patient soon recovered his strength—Surgeon *Allen F. Peck, 1st N. M., Ft. Stanton, N.M., Dec. 31, 1862.*[21]

Note again the surgeon's assumption that if one event follows another, the two must be related. In this case, he concludes that, because his patient's chest pain was relieved after a blister was raised, the blister was responsible for the relief. Many of the "medications" used at this time caused bodily fluids to exit the body, via repeated bowel movements, vomiting, sweating, blistering, copious nasal discharges, urination, removal of blood, and, unique to mercury, excessive salivation. The rationale was that an imbalance in the body's four humors—blood, black bile, yellow bile and phlegm—caused illnesses. By removing bodily fluids in any of several ways, balance could be restored. It is fascinating that this humoral theory of disease was accepted, essentially unchallenged, since the time of Hippocrates (460-370 B.C.), and that with all the leeching and other means of bleeding people, no one ever saw black or yellow bile or phlegm—just red blood, and yet did not question this ancient tenet. The human leech is shown in Figure 3.

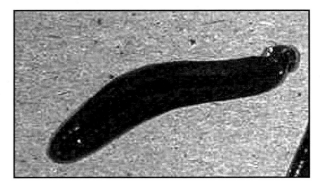

Figure 3. The human leech was used to remove blood believed by some surgeons to contain substances that caused sickness in the soldiers serving in the Civil War. *Courtesy of Peter Brodfuehrer, Ph.D.*

Results of using mercury in these four diseases are shown in the table on the facing page.

Table I. Outcomes of Treatment with Mercury[22-26]

Dysentery

3 of 94 Cases were given mercury; 2 of these 3 died, with a mortality of 67%

17 of 91 not given mercury died, with a mortality of 19%

Typhoid fever

9 of 51 given mercury; 0 died, with a mortality of 0%

9 of 42 not given mercury died, with a mortality of 21%

35 of 68 given mercury; 7 died, with a mortality of 20%

6 of 33 not given mercury died, with a mortality of 18%

Malaria

18 of 52 given mercury; 2 died, with a mortality of 11%

7 of 34 not given mercury died, with a mortality of 21%

Pneumonia

5 of 18 given mercury; 1 died, with a mortality of 20%

4 of 13 not given mercury died, with a mortality of 31%

It is interesting that in the first group of patients with typhoid fever, as well as those with malaria or pneumonia, more soldiers died in the groups not given mercury than in the ones that were. This could be interpreted as evidence that mercury was a successful treatment for some patients with typhoid and for malaria and pneumonia, but not for dysentery. What is not known is other information, such as why certain patients were selected to receive mercury, and others not. Was mercury used, for example, only in patients with mild illness who would have recovered anyway? Until the era of controlled trials of medications in which patients with a given disease, having the same degree of severity, are assigned randomly to the drug being tested or to a placebo, treatment was often based on the experience of an individual surgeon or on guidelines drawn up by several surgeons, which again were supported by experience and not on experimental proof of efficacy.

Preparations of mercury. Two sources of information about mercury available to surgeons, during their training in medical school or as practicing physicians in the decade before the Civil War, are *Joseph Carson's Materia Medica of 1851*[27] and Alfred Stillé's *Therapeutics and Materia Medica* (1860).[28] Freeman Bumstead's chapter on venereal diseases in Hammond's *Military Medical and Surgical Essays Prepared for the U.S. Sanitary Commission* of 1864 provided useful information during the war.[29] The following are the forms used most commonly, along with their preparation, indication for use and dose:

Chapter VIII

Blue pills; mercurial pills. These are made from "an ounce of mercury rubbed with an ounce and a half of confection of roses, and then beaten with half an ounce of powdered liquorice root."[30] Dose, for the bowels [as a cathartic] is 5 to 10 grains [300 to 600 milligrams] once; dose for the system, as an alterative [altering the course of a disease] is 1,2, or 3 grains [60, 120, 180 mg] repeated at intervals.[31]

Mercury with chalk. This is used as an antacid or an alterative. The "dose, ...for adults, grs [grains] V to XX [300 to 1200 mg]." "Irritation of the stomach [is] sometimes produced by it."[31]

Calomel; mild chloride of mercury; mercurous chloride. Stillé describes the laborious and dangerous synthesis of calomel:

> Take of mercury, *four pounds*; Sulphuric acid, *three pounds*; chloride of sodium, *a pound and a half*; distilled water, *a sufficient quantity*. Boil two pounds of the mercury with the Sulphuric acid, until a dry, white mass is left. Rub this, when cold, with the remainder of the mercury, in an earthenware mortar, until they are thoroughly mixed. Then add the chloride of sodium and rub it with the other ingredients till all the globules disappear; afterwards sublime [convert the solid to a gas without passing through a liquid phase]. Reduce the sublimed matter to a very fine powder, and wash it frequently with boiling distilled water, till the washings afford no precipitate upon the addition of solution of ammonia; then dry it.[32]

Carson advocates its use "to improve the secretions, to promote the activity of and unload the liver, ...gr ½ to j [30 to 60 mg] may be given two or three times daily."[33]

Compound cathartic pills. Stillé describes preparation of these:

> Compound extract of colocynth [dried bitter apple], ...*half an ounce*; extract of jalap [dried root of *Exogonium jalapa*], calomel, each *three drachms [180 grains]*; gamboge [gum-resin from *Garcinia hanburyi*], in powder, *two scruples [40 grains]*. Mix them together; then with water form a mass, to be divided into one hundred and eighty pills. Dose, from *two* to *four* pills.[34]

Corrosive chloride of mercury; mercuric chloride; bichloride of mercury; corrosive sublimate. Stillé wrote:

> Take of mercury, *two pounds*; sulphuric acid, *three pounds*; chloride of sodium, *a pound and a half*. Boil the mercury with the sulphuric acid until a white dry mass is left. Rub this, when cold, with the chloride of sodium, in an earthenware mortar; then sublime with a gradually increasing heat.[34]

Carson defines its mechanism of action when very small doses are prescribed: "In minimum doses, it acts as an alterative...." The dose is gr 1/16 to 1/12.[35] This form of mercury is very soluble and would be quite toxic in any but tiny doses.

Mercurial ointment; ammoniated mercury. This is made "by rubbing together two pounds of mercury, twenty-three ounces of lard, and an ounce of suet."[34]

Ammoniated mercury ointment; Of this Carson says it is an "irritant and poisonous." "Used externally...[as an ointment]...." It can also be applied as "the dry powder."[33]

Iodide of mercury; protoiodide of mercury. Bumstead recommends "gr X [600 mg] in 20 pills. One [30 mg per pill] after each meal [to treat syphilis]."[35] Carson says that the dose is 15 to 60 mg in pill form, but does not identify situations suitable for its use. He points out that it is also used externally in ointment form.[33]

Red iodide of mercury; biniodide of mercury. "Acrid and poisonous in over-doses; in minute doses, alterative. Dose, gr 1/16, in pill, or compound solution. Used extensively in the form of an ointment."[33]

The particulars of mercury today. *Stedman's Medical Dictionary* characterizes it as: "A dense liquid metallic element, atomic no. 80, atomic wt. 200.59." It is also called hydrargyrum or quicksilver. "Some salts and organic mercurials are used medicinally; care must be followed with its handling." It still is "used in thermometers, barometers, manometers, and other scientific instruments."[36] About the way the mercury-filled modern thermometers work, the same source states this instrument is a:

> Sealed vacuum tube containing mercury, which expands with heat and contracts with cold, its level accordingly rising or falling in the tube, with the exact degree of variation of level being indicated by a scale.

The clinical thermometer is a self-registering thermometer in which:

> Only the highest temperature is registered, usually by a steel bar above the column of mercury or by a segment of the mercury separated from the main column by a bubble of air; after the maximum temperature is registered, the bar or segment of mercury remains in place as the column of mercury contracts.[37]

History of the clinical thermometer. In 1714 Gabriel Daniel Fahrenheit, a German physicist living in Holland, developed the thermometer and the scale (boiling point of water being 212°) that bears his name.[38] In 1717 this same scientist introduced the mercury thermometer, replacing those that previously used alcohol.

Mercury was superior because it had a more uniform expansion rate and a much wider temperature range. In 1724 Fahrenheit introduced a scale with zero as the temperature of snow mixed with ammonium chloride, 32° as the freezing point of water, 96° as "the mouth temperature of a healthy human being," and 212° as the boiling point of water.[39]

Not until 1868 was the first work on clinical thermometry (measurement of the temperature in healthy and in sick humans) published, and that was done in Germany.[40] In 1870 the modern self-registering thermometer was introduced by Thomas Clifford Allbutt, in the British and Foreign Medical-Chirurgical Review.[41] Thermometers used by surgeons serving in the Civil War had to be read while the thermometer was held in place, usually in the armpit. Since they were not self-registering, when the surgeon removed the thermometer, the temperature dropped at once to the temperature of ambient air. One example of such an instrument is shown in Figure 4. In Figure 5 is a clinical mercury thermometer typical of those in use today.

Figure 4. Mercury thermometer of the Civil War period. The bend was necessary because the thermometer had to be read while the thermometer remained in the patient's armpit. The self-registering thermometer had not yet been invented. *Courtesy, Mütter Museum, College of Physicians of Philadelphia.*

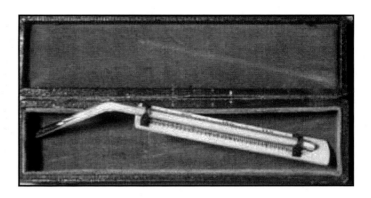

Figure 5. Self-registering thermometer, able to be read after being withdrawn from the measurement site in a patient. *Author's collection.*

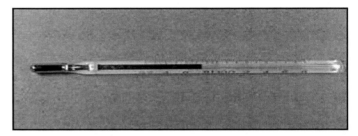

Contemporary medical thinking about mercury: what physicians—in England, in the U.S. in civilian practice, and in the army—thought about how mercury worked. John Beck, an American, states, in 1849:

> Except in the venereal disease, it was not until...the last century [1700s] that an extensive use was made of the preparations of mercury; and it was then, that it was introduced into the treatment of inflammatory complaints. This practice took its rise in this country, and to the enterprize [sic] of American physicians is mainly due the credit of the general introduction of this powerful agent into practical medicine.[42]

Beck credits its use to "an eccentric but eminent physician, of Boston," Dr. William Douglass, and relates the circumstances that led to its introduction for other than sexually transmitted disease:

> An epidemic called the *putrid sore throat*, ...commenced its career in May, 1735, at Kingston, ...New Hampshire. It was in attempting to arrest the ravages of this dreadful epidemic, that mercury appears to have been first introduced into the treatment of inflammatory complaints, ...[by] Dr. Douglass.... The preparation of mercury which he used was calomel [mercurous chloride]. The following is his language...[in 1736]. 'Where nature required any assistance, the principal intentions were with regard to the...[rash and ulcers] in the throat. Any affection in the throat does frequently produce a natural ptyalism [increase in saliva]; *mercurials* used with discretion, are a kind of specific in such like ulcers..., and...here they moistened the throat and mouth, stopt [sic] the spreading of the...[ulcers], and promoted the casting off of the sloughs [membranes].... Amongst all the preparations, *calomel* answered best, the gentle vomiting, or few stools that it occasioned in some, did not confound the natural course of the...[disease].'[42]

Beck explains that after its efficacy in the 1735 epidemic, mercury was used to treat other diseases and was given in different quantities, depending on the reason for its use:

> In consequence of the reputation which calomel thus acquired in the treatment of this disease, it came very naturally to be resorted to in other inflammatory diseases, and accordingly, about the middle of the last century, it was in common use in pleurisy, pneumonia, [and] inflammatory rheumatism.... The common practice was to give it in large doses, when used as a cathartic; and when given as an alterant, or to affect the system, in doses of one or two grains.[42]

Dr. Beck's assessment, interestingly, is borne out by modern pharmacology. In high doses, mercury is a laxative (cathartic) and passes through the gastrointestinal tract so quickly that little can be absorbed. Small doses in the range of one or two grains (60 to 120 mg), however, are absorbed and can cause the loss of a large quantity of urine (diuresis) and the production of copious saliva (ptyalism). These are two of the ways physicians of the Civil War period thought they were ridding the body of harmful substances, thereby restoring the balance of the four humors, as discussed under *Pneumonia*, above.

Putative mechanism of action of mercury. P.W. Ellsworth, M.D., in 1845 writes, "Mercurial preparations, and calomel in particular, probably owe...their curative power to...diminishing the...fibrine [in the blood, thereby]...leaving...[the circulation] to operate naturally, being relieved of...[this burden]...."[43] Alfred Stillé, M.D., in 1860, views mercury as an alterative [altering the course of a disease], that acts either "on the humors, diluting and therefore rendering their movements more easy and unobstructed, ...[or by affecting] the solids, modifying their tone, contractility, elasticity...and thus enabling them to circulate the fluids more rapidly and freely."[44]

Dr. S.O. Habershon, Fellow of the Royal College of Physicians and senior assistant physician and lecturer on *materia medica* and therapeutics at Guy's Hospital, London, reviews the beliefs of eight authorities on mercury, in 1840:

1. Dr. Wilson Philip:

    "Mercury, like other agents, possesses the *sedative* as well as the *stimulant* property; and its sedative properties appear to be wholly exerted...from its removing some cause of irritation."

2. Dr. Billing:

    It is a tonic. "By its specific action on the capillaries, it causes them to contract."

3. Dr. Dunglison:

    Mercury is an "*eutrophic*, a promoter of healthy nutrition...."

4. Dr. Pereira:

    It is a spanoemic, "an agent which impoverishes the blood."

Chapter VIII

5. Dr. Alison:

> That calomel and opium, used in moderation, is a useful medicine in many internal inflammations is granted by all, because the soothing effects of the opium are often desirable, and the calomel is one of the simplest means by which some of the injurious effects of opium may be corrected; but the main question, ...[regarding] mercury, is this—Do the symptoms of inflammatory diseases subside more rapidly, and more certainly, when the mercury has affected the mouth, than without that occurrence? And on this point observations are somewhat at variance. ... And as to the treatment of pneumonia, he tells us that, 'no reliance can be placed on the specific effect of mercury in preventing or resolving the... [diseased] lungs.'

6. Dr. Watson:

> [Favors] the idea that 'mercury tends to equalize the circulation; that by causing the blood to be distributed in larger quantity than common upon several surfaces at the same time, it obviates...its excessive congestion or accumulation in any one organ.' He...graphically describes it as 'a very potent, but two-edged weapon.' 'That it has a loosening effect upon certain textures; that it works by pulling down parts of the building.' But that 'the great remedial property of mercury is that of stopping...[the formation of certain fluids, like lymph]; of bridling...inflammation; and if we, in our turn, could always bridle and limit...mercury itself, it would be a still more valuable resource.' To the latter part of this quotation we give hearty assent, but...instead of stopping, we have very often seen the...[formation] of lymph increase [,] during its action.

7. Dr. Barlow:

> "By its action on the glands, 'it causes an increased flow of blood to...organs....' "

8. Dr. Neligan: In his discourse he concludes that the use of all of these names means that the mechanism by which mercury acts is not understood at all! Dr. Neligan:

> Mercury is a special stimulant, "comprising alteratives and specifics. The term *alterative* is one very frequently used to describe the effects produced by small doses of mercury; namely, that the medicine is given, no very marked effect is produced, but the alteration for the better has...[resulted]. This cluster of names—sedative, stimulant, tonic, special stimulant, eutrophic, alterative, spanoemic, resolvent are, of themselves, indication of the limited extent of our knowledge, as to the precise mode of action of a drug, perhaps more extensively used than any other.[45]

Until and unless these suppositions could be tested experimentally, the mechanism of action of mercury would remain unknown.

Toxic effects of mercury. In order to understand these, the way in which mercury interacts with the human body (its pharmacology) must be reviewed. In order to be absorbed into the body when given by mouth, mercury must be available in a form that dissolves in the intestinal contents (soluble). Mercury such as calomel (mercurous chloride; $HgCl$) is relatively insoluble. Some forms of mercury undergo oxidation to become soluble, absorbable compounds. In suitable vehicles, mercurials may also be absorbed through normal skin. Within a few hours mercury is found in human tissues in decreasing concentration in: pancreas, kidney, liver, spleen, blood, bone marrow, lining of the upper airways and mouth, intestinal wall (especially the colon), skin, salivary glands, heart, skeletal muscle, brain, and lung. Excretion (the body ridding itself) of mercury starts immediately after absorption, mainly by the kidney, colon, bile, and saliva. "Most of the mercury is excreted within 6 days after administration, but traces may be detected for months, even years."[46]

Acute mercury poisoning usually results from oral ingestion of mercury, but also may occur from topically applied mercurial ointment. When mercuric chloride ($HgCl_2$; corrosive chloride of mercury) is ingested, precipitation of the lining of the mouth, throat, and stomach occurs, causing an ashen-gray appearance of these linings, instead of the normal red color. Intense pain in the affected tissues results, which is aggravated by vomiting. However, vomiting is protective; if the stomach is quickly and effectively emptied, the patient's chance for survival is much greater. If a high concentration of mercury reaches the lining of the small intestine, severe, profuse, bloody diarrhea soon occurs. Shreds of intestinal lining can be seen in the stool; severe shock and death may result.[47]

In 1851 Joseph Carson describes several complications after mercury is administered in doses less than those causing the immediately fatal condition described above. "When the impression is inordinate, or in peculiar constitutions, the entire...system becomes so affected as to assume a morbid condition, and an especial disease is engrafted upon the system, called *Morbus Mercurialis*...." He lists these as excessive salivation, erythema mercurialis [red rash], febris mercurialis [fever], excessive general prostration, and nervous perturbation [hyperactivity, as in the Mad Hatter in Lewis Carroll's *Alice in Wonderland*]. Mental disturbances were a known consequence of being a hatter, caused by the toxic effects of mercury used in hat manufacture. Carson is insightful in his observation that there is a "difference in the susceptibility of individuals" to these complications.[48] The most extreme manifestation of mercurial toxicity is salivation, or ptyalism. Dr. Alfred Stillé, in 1860, writes this description:

> Of all the usual effects of the full mercurial operation, salivation is the most striking. ...the salivary glands also become swollen and tender, and their secretion [saliva] is augmented and of a ropy consistence [sic], ...and of a penetrating taste and smell. Several pints of it may be discharged in the course of twenty-four hours. When mercurial salivation is excessive, these symptoms sometimes reach distressing degree. The swelling of the mouth and tongue renders...[swallowing] and speech difficult, if not impossible; extensive ulcers...attack the gums, cheeks, and...[back of the throat], and, in healing, may cause permanent adhesions of contiguous parts; oedema [swelling] of the...[throat] may occur, the breath becomes insufferably fetid, the teeth loosen and fall out, and caries [cavities] may attack the remaining teeth, and even the maxillary [upper jaw] bones.[48]

Habershon, in 1840, notes that the quantity of mercury required to produce salivation is sometimes very small and that a "Dr. Christison mentions an instance in which two grains of calomel produced fatal salivation...."[49] Dr. Frank Netter illustrated masterfully the toxic effects of mercury in the mouth in 1959.[50]

Gangrene of the jaw may occur after salivation, with even six grains of calomel. Woodward quotes a report by a Dr. A. Campbell, in 1834:

Chapter VIII

> The patient, a boy 14 years old, suffering with malarial fever, took a purgative dose of three grains of calomel and eight of colocynth [dried bitter apple], followed next morning by a drachm of compound powder of jalap [dried root used as a laxative]. This operated freely, and was repeated with the same result two days afterwards. Two days later the mouth began to swell, and mercurial foetor [foul breath], ulceration and gangrene of the gums, palate and lips followed, from which the patient died fifteen days after the first dose.[51]

This complication prompted Union Surgeon General Hammond to ban calomel from the supply table of the Union Army, as will be seen later.

A severe blistering rash is another complication of mercury poisoning. Called *hydrargyria maligna*, it is described vividly in this account by Dr. George Alley in 1810:

> 1. The sense of burning on the surface is experienced to a very painful degree. 2. The actual heat of the skin becomes intense. 3. The soreness of the throat...is extreme. 4. The colour of the eruption is...[dark], rising sometimes even to purple; and there is considerable tumefaction [swelling] of the surface. 5. Vesicles [blisters] of a...[large] size...precede desquamation [shedding of the skin].
>
> The tumefaction of the surface is accompanied with a most painful burning sensation, as of blistering from fire. This is peculiarly distressing, immediately previous to desquamation, when the actual heat of the body is greatly increased, rising sometimes to 108° of Fahrenheit. About this period also, blisters even of considerable magnitude are formed; and, when they break, an acrimonious lymph is discharged. The...[blisters] are so numerous that the whole of the...[skin]...[separates] from the surface of the body, which is swollen.... As the disease advances, ...[liquid oozes] from the surface..., and acquires a most offensive odour. [The] odour [is so disagreeable] as to induce nausea in the patient himself, and those who approach near the bedside.
>
> The cuticle frequently scales off in very large pieces; and from the hand, especially, I have seen it to separate so entire as to resemble a glove.[52]

Still another adverse effect is "mercurial purging," described by Stillé, in his two-volume textbook, *Therapeutics and Materia Medica*, of 1860:

> This is not the direct effect of purgative doses of mercury, but is an affection in which, during the constitutional operation of the medicine, the alvine evacuations [stools] become at first feculent [foul smelling], thin, and greenish, and afterwards watery or frothy, and ale in color. There may be ten or fifteen of such stools in the course of twenty-four hours. At the same time there is a sense of fulness [sic] in the abdomen, tenderness on pressure in the epigastria [upper abdomen], and a dull...pain in the same region. The thirst is great, the mouth and skin dry, and the urine scanty. As the diarrhea augments, vomiting may be superadded, while the skin grows cool and the eyes are sunken and dark. The affection may terminate in gastric inflammation [irritation of the stomach].[53]

It is of interest that when given to treat dysentery, mercury did not appear to cause struc-

Figure 6. Specimen #115 of the Army Medical Museum, Medical Section, from Case 897. Colon of a soldier treated twice with mercury for dysentery. There are ulcers and a pseudomembrane typical of a patient with dysentery. *From* Medical and Surgical History of the War of the Rebellion (1861–1865), *Medical History, Part 2, Vol. 1. 1879: facing p. 454.*

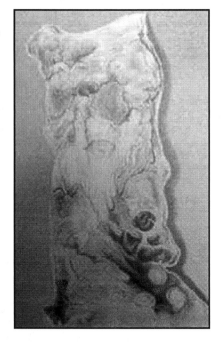

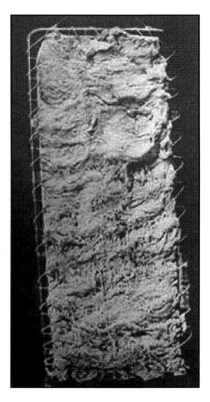

Figure 7. Colon from Case 893 (see page 88), showing ulcers and a pseudomembrane indistinguishable from those in Figure 6. *From* Medical and Surgical History of the War of the Rebellion (1861–1865), *Medical History, Part 2, Vol. 1. 1879: facing p. 446.*

tural changes in the large bowel. Figure 6 exhibits the colon of Private Taylor W. Glascow, who received two courses of mercury. In Figure 7 is a specimen of large bowel from a soldier who died of dysentery for whom mercury was not prescribed.

The Hammond imbroglio. Below is the document signed by Surgeon General William A. Hammond, removing one form of mercury—calomel—from the Union Army's supply table:

Circular No. 6. Surgeon General's Office, *Washington, D. C.,* May 4, 1863.

I. From the reports of medical inspectors and the sanitary reports to this office, it appears that the administration of calomel has so frequently been pushed to excess by military surgeons as to call for prompt steps by this office to correct this abuse; an abuse the melancholy effects of which, as officially reported, have exhibited themselves not only in innumerable cases of profuse salivation, but in the not infrequent occurrence of mercurial gangrene [of the

Chapter VIII

jaw]. It seeming impossible in any other manner to properly restrict the use of this powerful agent, it is directed that it be struck from the supply table, and that no further requisitions for this medicine be approved by medical directors. This is done with the more confidence as modern pathology has proved the impropriety of the use of mercury in very many of those diseases in which it was formerly unfailingly administered.

II. The records of this office having conclusively proved that diseases prevalent in the army may be treated as efficiently without tartar emetic as therewith, and the fact of its remaining upon the supply table being a tacit invitation to its use, tartar emetic is also struck from the supply table of the army. No doubt can exist that more harm has resulted from the misuse of both these agents, in the treatment of disease, than benefit from their proper administration.

W. A. Hammond, *Surgeon General*.[54]

Examination of supplies purchased and manufactured during the war by the Medical Department of the Army reveals that the Union Army bought 8,760 pounds of calomel alone, as well as 488,447 *dozen* compound cathartic pills, each containing 60 mg of calomel. As Surgeon J. S. Billings, U.S.A., says, "This quantity is altogether…more than three and a half…million scruple (avoirdupois, 10 grains, or 600 milligram) doses of calomel issued."[55] Not affected by Hammond's order were the 4,330 pounds of mercury with chalk bought or manufactured by the army, because it was prepared with elemental mercury, not calomel, which is mercurous chloride.[56] Use of mercury by the Confederate Army was similar. A single Confederate medical laboratory at Columbia, South Carolina, produced in one quarter 2,005 pounds of mercurial-pill mass.[57]

Twenty-six days after Circular No. 6 was issued, several physicians in Cincinnati adopted the following resolution, published in the *Cincinnati Medical and Surgical News*: "Resolved, that the removal of W.A. Hammond from his position as Surgeon General would meet the approbation of the profession, be of advantage to our soldiers and creditable to the government."[58] Many of the signatories to this resolution had observed patients in general hospitals and in the western armies and claimed not to have seen the abuses alluded to by Hammond. On June 2, 1863, during the 14th annual meeting of the American Medical Association in Chicago, a Dr. Lawson of Ohio offered this resolution:

In relation to order of the Surgeon General, prohibiting the use of calomel and antimony [tartar emetic is antimony potassium tartrate], in the Army, — Resolved, that a committee of one from each state represented in this association, be appointed to inquire into a recent order issued by the Surgeon General of the United States Army, in which the further supply of calomel and antimony is prohibited, and to report at as early a period as may be convenient, during the present session.[59]

On August 18, 1864, William A. Hammond was convicted in a court-martial and removed as Surgeon General of the Union Army, having served in that position since April 25, 1862. Of that proceeding we learn from *Reply of the judge advocate, John A. Bingham, to the defence [sic] of the accused, before a general court-martial for the trial of Brig. Gen. William A. Hammond, Surgeon General, U.S.A.*: "Of the many offences wherewith the accused stands charged, all, save one, are alleged violations of the statute entitled 'An act to reorganize and increase the medical department of the army,' approved April 16, 1862."

The charges were:

I. "Disorders and neglects to the prejudice of good order and military discipline."

II. "Conduct unbecoming an officer and a gentleman."

III. "Conduct to the prejudice of good order and military discipline."[60]

Officially these charges related to purchasing blankets of substandard quality for the army. Hammond's removal of two widely prescribed medications—calomel and antimony—from the Army supply table, however, figured prominently in the decision to court-martial him. Actually the seeds of Hammond's dismissal were probably sown as early as the month after his confirmation as Surgeon General, when he and Secretary of War Edwin McMasters Stanton engaged in the first of many caustic verbal disputes.[61] Stanton's decision to oust Hammond became even more certain when his major supporter, Frederick Law Olmsted, left the U.S. Sanitary Commission on September 1, 1863.[62] On August 22, 1864, Joseph K. Barnes, M.D., was appointed Hammond's successor.

Mercurials continued to be prescribed for 40 years following the Civil War, as shown in this entry from *Merck's Manual of the Materia Medica*, of 1899:

Mercury, U. S. P. Preparations:

    A. Mass (33 percent).
    B. Mercury with Chalk.
    C. Ointment (50 percent).
    D. Plaster (18 percent).
    E. Ammoniac and Mercury Plaster (30 percent Hg).
    F. Mercury Dichloride (Corrosive Mercuric Chloride). Dose: 1/32 to 1/12 grain.
    G. Mercury Chloride (Mercurous Chloride, Calomel).
    H. Mercury Iodide, Red (Mercury Biniodide). Dose 1/16 to 1/4 grain, in pills.
    I. Mercury Iodide, Yellow (Proto-Iodide). Dose 1/2 to 2 grain.
    J. Mercury Oxide, Black (Hahnemann's Soluble Mercury). Dose 1/2 to 3 grain.
    K. Mercury Oxycyanide. White powder. Soluble in water. Antiseptic; said superior as antiseptic dressing to mercuric chloride because more active as germicide and less easily absorbed. Applied in 0.6% solution to wounds and in surgical operations.
    L. Mercury Sulphate (Turpeth Mineral). Dose: emetic 2–5 grain; alterative 1/4 to 1/2 grain in pills or powder.
    M. Mercury Salicylate. White powder; about 59% mercury. Uses: *External*, chancre, gonorrhea…; 1% powder or ointment; *injection* in urethra, 1–5% water. Reported easily borne by the stomach, and to produce no salivation. Dose: 1/3–1 grain.
    N. Mercury Tannate Merck. Greenish-gray powder; about 50% mercury. Antisyphilitic. Dose 1-2 grain, in pills.
    O. Mercury Ammonium Chloride. White Precipitate; Ammoniated Mercury. Not used internally. Preparation: Ointment, 10%.[63]

Mercurials still in medical use today are shown in Appendix VI. As late as 1975, mercury was still used as a diuretic. It was the only such medication during the preceding thirty years.

The soldiers commonly referred to blue mercury pills as thunderclappers, because of their relief of constipation. Interestingly, that term antedated the Civil War, having been used at least as early as 1803, by the Corps of Discovery (the Lewis and Clark expedition):

Since the men were plagued with gastrointestinal problems from their nearly all-meat diet and from drinking muddy river water, the pills—which were nearly 60% mercury were freely dispensed. While they may not have cured any illnesses, the thunderclappers have served archaeologists well: traces of mercury remain in the soil along the Corps of Discovery's route, and some expedition campsites have been identified by excavating corps latrines.[64]

Chapter VIII References

1. Stillé A. *Therapeutics and Materia Medica*, Vol. II. Philadelphia: Blanchard and Lea; 1860: 772
2. *Medical and Surgical History of the Civil War*. Wilmington, NC: Broadfoot Publishing; Vol. I; 1990: 637, 710. Hereafter *MSHCW*
3. *MSHCW* Vol. III; 1990: 45–65, 101–257
4. *Ibid.*, 146
5. *Medical and Surgical History of the War of the Rebellion (1861–65)*. Washington, DC: Government Printing Office, Medical History, Part 2, Vol. 1, 1879: 446. Hereafter *MSHWR (1861–1865)*
6. Webster's New Twentieth Century Dictionary of the English Language Unabridged, 2nd edition, New York: World Publishing Co.; 1964: 843
7. Netter FH. *Ciba Collection of Medical Illustrations, Digestive System*, Vol. 3, Part II. West Caldwell, NJ: Ciba; 1962: 154
8. *MSHCW* Vol. I; 1990: 637, 710
9. *MSHCW* Vol. V; 1990: 216–249
10. *Ibid.*, 218
11. *Ibid.*, 219
12. Woodward JJ. *Outline of the chief camp diseases of the United States Armies*; Philadelphia: J.B. Lippincott & Co., 1863. Repub.: New York: Hafner Pub. Co.; 1964: 322
13. *MSHCW* Vol. I: 637, 710
14. *MSHCW* Vol. V; 1990: 112–119; 131–144
15. Stillé A. *Therapeutics and Materia Medica*, Vol. II. Philadelphia: Blanchard and Lea, 1860: 772
16. *MSHCW* Vol. V; 1990: 112
17. *Ibid.*, 113
18. Morton L T, Moore R J. *A Chronology of Medicine and Related Sciences*. Brookfield, VT: Ashgate; 1997: 41
19. *MSHCW* Vol. I; 1990: 639, 711
20. *MSHCW* Vol. VI; 1990: 752–755
21. *Ibid.*, 752
22. *MSHCW* Vol. III; 1990: 45–65
23. *MSHCW* Vol. V; 1990: 216–229
24. *Ibid.*, 229–249
25. *Ibid.*, 112–119
26. *MSHCW* Vol. VI; 1990: 752–755
27. Dorwart BB. *Carson's Materia Medica of 1851: An Annotation*. Bala Cynwyd, PA; WVD Press; 2003: 45–49
28. Stillé A. *Therapeutics and Materia Medica*, Vol. II. Philadelphia: Blanchard and Lea; 1860: 772–75
29. Bumstead FJ. Chap. XVII, Venereal Diseases, in *Military Medical and Surgical Essays Prepared for the U.S.S.C.*, ed. Hammond WA; Philadelphia: J.B. Lippincott & Co.; 1864: 549
30. Stillé A. *Therapeutics and Materia Medica*, Vol. II. Philadelphia: Blanchard and Lea; 1860: 772–775

31. Dorwart BB. *Carson's Materia Medica of 1851: An Annotation.* Bala Cynwyd, PA: WVD Press; 2003: 45–49
32. Stillé A. *Therapeutics and Materia Medica,* Vol. II. Philadelphia: Blanchard and Lea; 1860: 772–775
33. Dorwart BB. *Carson's Materia Medica of 1851: An Annotation.* Bala Cynwyd, PA: WVD Press; 2003: 45–49
34. Stillé A. *Therapeutics and Materia Medica,* Vol. II. Philadelphia: Blanchard and Lea; 1860: 772–775
35. Bumstead FJ. Chap. XVII, Venereal Diseases, in *Military Medical and Surgical Essays Prepared for the U.S.S.C.*, ed. Hammond WA; Philadelphia: J.B. Lippincott & Co.; 1864: 549
36. *Stedman's Medical Dictionary,* 26th ed. Baltimore: Williams & Wilkins; 1995: 1091
37. *Ibid.,* 1802
38. Desmond K. *A Timetable of Inventions and Discoveries,* New York: M. Evans & Co.; 1986: 1714
39. Turner GL´E. *Scientific Instruments 1500–1900.* London: Philip Wilson Publishers; 1998: 111
40. Wunderlich C. *Das Verhalten der Eigenwärme in Krankheiten [The Temperature in Diseases]*: 1868
41. Morton LT, Moore RJ. *A Chronology of Medicine and Related Sciences.* Brookfield, VT, Ashgate Publishing Co.; 1997: 304, 312
42. Beck J. *Essays on Infant therapeutics: to which are added Observations on Ergot, and an Account of the Origin of the use of Mercury in Inflammatory Complaints.* New York: W. E. Dean; 1849: 110–117
43. Ellsworth PW. On the Modus operandi of Medicines, *The Boston Medical and Surgical Journal.* 1845; 32: 372
44. Stillé A. *Therapeutics and Materia Medica,* Vol. II. Philadelphia: Blanchard and Lea; 1860: 767
45. Habershon SO. *On the injurious effects of mercury in the treatment of disease.* London: John Churchill; 1840: 15–24
46. Goodman L, Gilman A. *The Pharmacological Basis of Therapeutics,* 5th ed. New York: Macmillan Publishing Co., Inc.; 1975: 823–825
47. *Ibid.,* 935–936
48. Carson J. *Synopsis of the Course of Lectures on Materia Medica and Pharmacy, Delivered in the University of Pennsylvania.* Philadelphia: Blanchard and Lea; 1851: 45–49
48. Stillé A. *Therapeutics and Materia Medica,* Vol. II. Philadelphia: Blanchard and Lea; 1860: 785–86
49. Habershon SO. *On the injurious effects of mercury in the treatment of disease.* London: John Churchill; 1840: 8–9
50. Netter. FH. *Ciba Collection of Medical Illustrations, Digestive System,* Vol. 3, Part I West Caldwell, NJ; 1959: 116.
51. Campbell A. Fatal Effects of Calomel. *The India Jour. of Med. Sci.,* Vol. I. 1834: 74, in *MSHCW,* Vol. IV; 1990: 723
52. Alley G. *Observations on the Hydrargyria; or that vesicular disease arising from the exhibition of mercury.* London: Whittingham and Rowland, for Longman, Hurst, Rees, and Orme; 1810: 29–32
53. Stillé A. *Therapeutics and Materia Medica,* Vol. II. Philadelphia: Blanchard and Lea; 1860: 792
54. *MSHCW* Vol. IV. 1990: 719
55. *Ibid.,* 722
56. *MSHCW,* Vol. VI. 1990: 966
57. Hasegawa GR, Hambrecht FT. *The Confederate Medical Laboratories. South Med J.* 2003; 96: 1221–1230
58. Meeting of the Medical Profession Upon Surgeon General Hammond's Order No. 6. *Cincinnati Med. and Surg. News,* Vol. IV. 1863: 217
59. *Ibid.,* 204–216
60. *Reply of the judge advocate, John A. Bingham, to the defence of the accused, before a general court–martial for the trial of Brig. Gen. William A. Hammond, Surgeon General, USA.* Washington: Govt. Printing Office; 1864: 2–3
61. Rutkow IM. *Bleeding Blue and Gray: Civil War Surgery and the Evolution of American Medicine.* New York: Random House; 2005: 119
62. *Ibid,* 279–280
63. *Merck's Manual of the Materia Medica,* 1ST ed. New York: Merck and Co.; 1899: 49–50
64. *Smithsonian.* 2004 (June): 22

Chapter IX.

Mercury after Venus:

The Use of Mercury to Treat Syphilis

Although case reports of soldiers who contracted syphilis are lacking, it is clear that many thousands of men had the disease. Between May 1861, and June 30, 1866, there were 73,382 cases recorded in white troops.[1] From June of 1864 to June 30 of 1866, 6,207 cases occurred in United States Colored Troops.[2]

In Chapter V, under *Syphilitic arthritis*, the natural history of this sexually transmitted disease was discussed, but a brief review is appropriate before exploring the world of the Civil War surgeon who was faced with treating it. The earliest manifestation, about three weeks after sexual exposure, is the ulcer (chancre), firm to the touch, usually on the penis, accompanied by swollen lymphatic glands in the groin (bubo). Secondary syphilis occurs if primary syphilis is not treated in a way that insures absorption of the medication into the body, since the infection spreads internally within hours or days of infection, even before the chancre appears. Occurring in the secondary stage are skin rash, mucous patches in the mouth, and swollen glands all over the body. In the next stage, the disease seems to disappear or be cured because there are no abnormalities when the patient is examined and he feels well. This so-called latent syphilis was not recognized until 1906, when Wassermann, Neisser, and Bruck introduced a blood test (the *Wassermann test*) to diagnose syphilis. Late (tertiary) syphilis, occurring years after the infection, may involve the aorta, brain and spinal cord. As early as 1822, A.L.J. Bayle described the dementia and impaired walking characteristic of tertiary syphilis of the brain and cord, but did not know what caused the entity. Proof of that awaited isolation of *Treponema pallidum*—the spirochete that causes syphilis—from the brain of a patient with syphilitic dementia in 1913 by Noguchi and Moore.

Medical thought of the time concerning the chancre. Dr. Freeman Bumstead, who wrote the chapter on venereal diseases in *Hammond's Military Medical and Surgical Essays prepared for the U. S. Sanitary Commission* in 1864, was a keen observer:

> The syphilitic chancre is: always derived from an infecting chancre.... Its first appearance often from one to five weeks after contagion. Characteristic Gland affection. —All the superficial inguinal ganglia [lymph glands] on one or both sides enlarged and indurated [firm]; distinct from each other, freely movable; painless, and rarely suppurate [discharge pus]. Prognosis. —A constitutional [throughout the patient's body] affection. Secondary symptoms, unless prevented or retarded by treatment, declare themselves in about six weeks from the appearance of the sore [chancre], and very rarely delay longer than three months.[3]

Bumstead then explains that treating the chancre alone is insufficient and cites the evidence on which his opinion is based:

> [A] chancre...is already the result of absorption of the virus and of infection of the constitution, and not a mere local disease; hence, ...its abortive treatment by destructive cauterization [caustic chemical applied to the chancre] is incapable of averting general syphilis; hence, also,...it should receive the same...treatment as...[generalized syphilis]. *Clinical experience confirms this view, since thorough destruction of a chancre six hours after its first appearance has failed to avert general symptoms.* [emphasis added]
>
> Experience also proves that the cicatrization [local destruction, scarring] of chancre...is hastened by the internal use of mercury. This sore, therefore, demands the same internal treatment as general syphilis.[4]

His treatment is mercury taken by mouth. He states, "No one form of mercurial is adapted to all cases," and lists several preparations as well as dosage and frequency of administration.[5] He does not, however, elaborate on when each should be used.

Other surgeons of the era disagree about the nature of the chancre and hence about the treatment of syphilis. One who believed that a caustic chemical applied to the chancre destroys it is Surgeon Isaac F. Galloupe, 17th Massachusetts Infantry. On February 20, 1863, he recommended, "Cauterization of the chancre..., followed by the continuous application of black wash [mercury oxide]." He said, "All cases thus treated recovered without secondary disease."[6] Perhaps Dr. Galloupe did not wait a sufficient period of time for secondary syphilitic symptoms to appear, or perhaps the rash and lymph node swelling were mild and the soldiers under his care did not report them at daily Surgeon's Call, where the sick appeared for treatment.

Assistant Surgeon P. W. Randall, 1st California Infantry, Fort Bragg, California, favored treatment by mouth and by cauterization of the chancre. On New Year's Day in 1863, Surgeon Randall wrote, "For syphilis I use mercurial and saline [Epsom salt solution is one example] purges [cathartics], rest, low diet, iodide of potassium and bichloride of mercury, with caustic to chancres...."[6] Surgeon Ezra Read, 21st Indiana Infantry, Baltimore, Maryland, September 5, 1861, advocated mercury administered in still another way—by fumigation:

> For many years I have pursued the method of treatment by mercurial fumigation, which deposits the mercury upon the surface of the body when in a state of perspiration induced by the heated vapor of water surrounding the patient confined in a close and air-tight bath. This treatment is commended to our consideration because it eradicates the disease in a shorter period of time than is required by the internal use of mercury; moreover, when thus applied the constitutional [poisonous effects in the patient]...of the mercury are under satisfactory control.[6]

Note that all these methods are based on the experience of the individual surgeon, and not on any experimental information. None of the four—Bumstead, Galloupe, Randall, or Read—advocated salivating the patient with syphilis. For many doctors, however, salivation was thought to be necessary for treating that disease.

As early as the 1600s, Thomas Sydenham described salivation, and believed it must occur if syphilis were to be cured. To treat the French pox [the English term for syphilis], he used "salivation with mercury," by mixing lard (2 oz.) plus 1 oz. of quicksilver [another term for mercury] that the sick anoints:

> With his own hands his arms, thighs, and legs, three nights following.... When the salivation is come to a due height, that is most commonly, when *two quarts is spit* in the space of a night and a day; or if the symptoms vanish, tho [sic] he spit less, which most commonly happens four days after the salivation comes to its height. ... But if the *salivation abate* before the symptoms disappear, it must be *heightened* by giving now and then a scruple [1/24th of an ounce] of *mercuris dulcis* (mercurous chloride; calomel) for a dose.[7] [emphasis added]

Definitive treatment of syphilis was not available until Ehrlich introduced Arsphenamine, or Salvarsan, an arsenic derivative, in 1909.[8]

In my research for this book I did not find any reference to a controlled study that provided evidence that mercury was effective for treating syphilis. The first *Merck Manual* of 1899 still listed mercury for treatment. Any possible effectiveness would have depended on mercury being more toxic to the syphilis organism than to its hosts.

Chapter IX References

1. *Medical and Surgical History of the Civil War*. Wilmington, NC: Broadfoot Publishing; Vol. VI. 1990:891; Hereafter *MSHCW*
2. *MSHCW* Vol. I. 1990: 710
3. Bumstead, FJ. Chap. XVII, Venereal Diseases, in *Military Medical and Surgical Essays prepared for the USSC*, ed. Hammond WA. Philadelphia: J. B. Lippincottand Co.; 1864: 540–541
4. *Ibid.*, 545–546
5. *Ibid.*, 549
6. *MSHCW*, Vol. VI. 1990: 892
7. Sydenham T. Mercurialization. In: Pechey J, ed. *The Whole Works of that excellent Physician, Dr. Thomas Sydenham*, 7th ed. London: M. Wellington; 1717: 258
8. Morton LT, Moore RJ. *A chronology of medicine and related Sciences*. Brookfield, VT: Ashgate; 1997: 755

Chapter X.

How did Civil War Surgeons Keep Current with the Medical Advances of their Day?

That they read foreign journals and applied recently-published medical information to the treatment of their patients is illustrated by the experience of Dr. A. P. Frick, surgeon of the 103rd Pennsylvania Infantry, who received his M.D. from the University of Pennsylvania School of Medicine in 1861. In January 1865, he removed a bullet from between the first and second ribs of Private Lemuel C. Slagle. His description of his postoperative care follows: "I then kept the entire chest enveloped in hot fomentations, changed every few hours, after a method at that time recommended in the German medical schools and published in our medical journals."[1]

Rutkow details the efforts of Confederate Surgeon General Samuel Preston Moore to insure continuing medical education of his surgeons:

> Due to the immensity of the hostilities, the meeting of medical societies and publication of professional journals and books were almost totally suspended. Moore undertook the task of keeping his medical officers informed of the progress within their profession. In August 1863 he organized the Association of Army and Navy Surgeons of the Confederate States. This group met regularly to hear reports on medical and surgical subjects. The Association promoted meetings and discussions of medical topics and functioned in the role of a surrogate medical society.
>
> It was under Moore's guidance that a number of projects were completed in the field of publishing. He encouraged the founding of the *Confederate States Medical and Surgical Journal* (January 1864-February 1865). The *Journal* presented interesting articles in the way of case reports, original investigations, reviews of foreign and American books and journals, listings of battlefields, and casualty reports. It was a widely read publication and its influence was greatly enhanced by the absence of any other such publication in the South. One of the most unusual Southern medical efforts enabled their officers to supply many of the army's drug needs through the preparation of medicines from plants indigenous to the Southern states. This prompted Moore to promote the publication and distribution of the 601-page *Resources of the Southern Fields and Forests: Medical, Economical, and Agricultural*, by Francis Peyre Porcher (1825-1895) in 1863. To more fully meet the needs of the field officer, Moore assigned a physician on his staff to prepare a collection of papers entitled *A Manual of Military Surgery*. This was published in October 1863 and served as a field manual on operative surgery.[2]

Chapter X

Dr. Joseph K. Barnes, who succeeded William Hammond as Surgeon General of the Union Army, disseminated recently-published medical information to his surgeons, when in March of 1864, he issued Circular No. 6 containing the paper, *Reflex Paralysis, the result of gunshot wounds*, by Silas Weir Mitchell, George Read Morehouse and William Williams Keen, Jr.[3] This publication grew out of case studies from one of the few specialty hospitals of the war, the Turner's Lane Hospital for neurologic diseases in Philadelphia. Barnes published the work "for the information of Medical Officers, in the belief that immediate and practical benefit may be derived from it."

Two prominent journals that published medical information were the *American Journal of the Medical Sciences* and the *Boston Medical and Surgical Journal*. The latter was formed by uniting the *Boston Medical Intelligencer* (1823–1828) with the *New England Medical Review and Journal* in 1828. One hundred years later it was renamed the *New England Journal of Medicine*, the title by which we know it today.

Another important journal that informed physicians was entitled *Transactions of the American Medical Association*. Amazingly, the American Medical Association (AMA), founded in 1847, began publishing the *Transactions of the AMA* only a few months later, in January of 1848. In the initial issue, that organization's Committee on Anesthetic Agents published a history of the introduction of ether and chloroform into the practice of surgery, described the action of these agents on patients, reported the results of surgeons in the Jefferson Medical College and the University of Pennsylvania School of Medicine who used them, and urged the continued accumulation of information as their use widened. Excerpts from these reports reveal much about the way ethical questions were raised concerning the use of new drugs and techniques, about the quality of information transmitted to doctors unfamiliar with new drugs, and about the types of surgical procedures in which the two anesthetics had been used.

An example of ethical considerations in using these new drugs [ether and chloroform were first described in English in the *London Medical Gazette* and in *Lancet* in 1847 by James Young Simpson] follows:

> The great question, which still divides medical opinion, is: can the annulling of pain by anaesthetic agents be produced without risk to life, or is the hazard so inconsiderable as to justify their employment in all cases where it is desirable to prevent the pain of surgical operations: In other words, do the risks and evils attendant upon the use of these agents in surgery, counterbalance the advantages afforded by exemption from pain, and to what extent and under what circumstances is it proper to use them?[4]

Physicians familiar with ether and chloroform recognized early that individual responses to these agents varied, and they publicized that information. Some patients were profoundly relieved of the pain incident to surgery; others were not. Surgeons noted that many patients remained awake but pain-free, while others were totally unaware of their surroundings during the operation. The general assessment, however, that anesthesia was a wondrous medical phenomenon was voiced in this pronouncement of the Anesthetics Committee of the American Medical Association:

> The fact is established, that certain ethereal vapors [and chloroform] when inhaled, will produce insensibility to pain, and that the most sensitive portions

of the living body may be divided by the knife of the surgeon, while his patient lies in a state of unconsciousness.[4]

Cases administered ether or chloroform by University of Pennsylvania faculty between October 20, 1847, and February 16, 1848, and the surgical procedures performed are tabulated in Appendix VII. Most of the operations were performed on structures close to the surface of the skin and large blood vessels and nerves would not have been encountered. The exceptions are, the amputation of a leg (#2) in the University of Pennsylvania series, and modification of an amputation stump (#1), amputation of a thigh (#5), and amputation of a leg (#41) in the Jefferson Medical College series. No deaths resulted from anesthesia; patient #41 expired from tetanus.[4] The status of the new anesthetic drugs is summed up thus:

> Although the anaesthetic agents have been open to liberal use in every part of the civilized world, ...the only conclusive instance of direct relation between an anaesthetic agent and death are two in number. Can antimony or opium show as clean a bill of health for the same period?[5]

There was no medical index to facilitate the location of current medical literature. The first one revolutionized the ability of physicians to exchange and share medical information. Not surprisingly, the large surgical and anesthesia experience of the Civil War provided the impetus to create such an index. Begun in 1880, it was printed by the Government Printing Office in Washington, D.C., and called the *Catalogue of the Library of the Surgeon General's Office U.S. Army*. It arranged publications by author and by subject, and was published subsequently as the *Index Medicus* until 2004, when it was supplanted by *PubMed* and other online resources.

International medical congresses, so important for continuing medical education and cross-fertilization of ideas about causes and treatments of diseases, were not held until 1867, when Paris hosted the first one.

Chapter X References

1. Davis AC. *Medical Affairs II, University of Pennsylvania Medical Alumni in the Civil War*. Philadelphia: University of Pennsylvania; Spring, 1961: 85
2. Rutkow I, in Moore SP. Regulations of the Confederate States of America Medical Department, in *Regulations for the Army of the Confederate States*. Richmond: Randolph; 1862. Repub. San Francisco: Norman publishing; 1992: Introduction, x–xii
3. *Medical and Surgical History of the Civil War*. Wilmington, NC: Broadfoot Publishing; Vol. XII, 1990: 729
4. *Trans AMA*, Vol. I. 1848: 176; 220–221
5. Bigelow HJ. Anaesthetic Agents, their mode of exhibition and physiological effects, *Trans AMA* Vol. I; 1848: 214

Chapter XI.

Implementing and Accruing Medical Knowledge: Not a Simple Matter

Sometimes there is an ancient body of work providing evidence that prophylaxis against a disease is effective. Such is the case with smallpox. The fascinating history of its prevention appears in Appendix VIII. Despite the recognized efficacy of vaccination (with cowpox scab material) or variolation (using smallpox scab matter) in the prevention of smallpox, the disease continued to be a problem during the Civil War. Among white Union troops 12,236 cases of smallpox were reported, of whom 4,717 died,[1] and 6,716 cases in U.S. Colored Troops, with 2,341 dead.[2] These numbers, from *Sickness and Mortality Reports* of the *Medical and Surgical History of the Civil War*, do not include soldiers cared for in either general or smallpox hospitals. Except for the Union Departments of the Northwest, of New Mexico, and of the Division of the Pacific, smallpox was present in every department during each year of the war.[3] How did that occur, when prophylaxis against smallpox was practiced in civilian populations since the turn of the nineteenth century?

Dr. Charles Smart, who succeeded Joseph Woodward as the author of the third medical volume of the *Medical and Surgical History of the War of the Rebellion (1861–1865)*, states that at the time of the war it was believed that "vaccination and revaccination…[would] preserve the individual from small-pox…." He sheds light on what actually happened among the troops regarding immunization or lack thereof. Although the Union Army regulations required every man to be vaccinated, only a "few of the State military authorities succeeded in fulfilling this requirement. For many years before the war there had been no systematic vaccination in the…[civilian] communities. Many of the volunteer troops had never been vaccinated…."[4] If troops requiring vaccination were exposed to a suspected case, "prompt isolation of suspected cases and the destruction by fire of all infected clothing, bedding and shelters were measures of the first consequence in restraining the spread of the disease until immunity was conferred by successful vaccination or revaccination."[5]

Among Confederate prisoners, there were reportedly 9,830 cases during the war with 2,624 dying of the disease.[6] What little is known about Walter Brice's war experience as Regimental Surgeon of the 9th Tennessee Infantry and 6th Tennessee Infantry concerns smallpox. When an epidemic of smallpox threatened the 1st, 6th, 9th and 27th Tennessee regiments just before the Battle of Missionary Ridge, Lieutenant William M. Cunningham of Brice's H [Avalanche] company was inoculated "with the virus of the smallpox and from the vaccine matter taken from his arm the whole brigade was vaccinated."[7] Another member of the Avalanche, D. W. Wicker, on route home to Tennessee at the end of the war, "contracted smallpox, which developed into a most virulent form the first day after reaching his home. He lost the sight of both eyes with that most dreadful disease. Smallpox was then…much dreaded."[8]

Major Brice encountered the fear of smallpox in the civilian population as well. In February of 1865, as he and others were returning from furlough in Troy, Tennessee, to their command in North Carolina the following incident occurred:

One very wet evening as they were tramping through Georgia they applied at a house for shelter from the inclemency of the night. The owner of the house said to them—'Gentlemen, we would gladly give you shelter but we have a fully developed case of smallpox in the house.' Dr. Brice promptly replied: 'It must be Providence that directed our steps to this place. I am a physician and surgeon and will treat the patient free of charge and give instructions for treatment which will insure his speedy recovery....' They were invited in....[9]

In the North, material for immunization was supplied by medical dispensaries in the form of crusts (scabs) obtained only from infants infected with smallpox. Crusts collected on the twelfth to thirteenth day from cattle with naturally-occurring cowpox were also supplied to the Union Army to confer immunity against smallpox.[10] However, many men tried vaccinating themselves with scabs from fellow soldiers and developed what appeared to be syphilis.[11] Since another name for syphilis is *great pox*, it is easy to imagine non-medical people confusing the two rashes and using the wrong one for self-inoculation. Several other instances of syphilis-like rashes were reported even when troops were vaccinated by a surgeon with either officially-sanctioned crusts or those of a patient with smallpox.[5] Fear of spreading or acquiring syphilis, or of developing an abscess or even sepsis, made some surgeons and many soldiers hesitant to carry out orders to vaccinate. We see that even when there is proof of effective prophylaxis in a serious disease like smallpox, execution of the science may be imperfect.

Another fundamental question, given that invisible living particles were thought to cause disease as early as the 16th century, is why it took so long before the germ theory was proven. When Girolamo Fracastoro (Fracastorius) wrote in 1546 that living creatures that could not be seen caused fevers,[12] the microscope had not been invented. Antoni van Leeuwenhoek (1632–1723) examined materials under his microscope, and observed moving, living little animals (animalcules). Some of these were bacteria, which he described and illustrated in 1684.[13] He did not, however, study diseased persons or animals, these bacteria being normal residents of his mouth. Even when the blood of people with disease was examined under the microscope, observations were not necessarily translated into useful applications. In 1658 Athanasius Kircher, in his *Scrutinium*, saw that the blood of patients with plague was filled with a "countless brood of worms not perceptible to the naked eye." He believed "animalculae" to be the cause of some infectious diseases.[14] Without experimentation, however, he could not prove it.

In 1850 Pierre François Olive Rayer (1793–1867) did so with anthrax. He inoculated "anthrax-infected sheep blood into other sheep and saw the anthrax bacillus (*B. anthracis*) in the blood of the infected sheep...,"[15] and published his results. Fifteen years later Casimir Joseph Davaine (1812–1882) showed that anthrax could also be transmitted to horses, cows, guinea pigs and mice, and that characteristic rod-shaped structures appeared in their blood 4 to 5 hours before death.[16] Not, however, until Robert Koch saw bacteria under the microscope in animals with anthrax, isolated those bacteria, injected only the anthrax bacteria into uninfected animals and produced anthrax in them, then recovered anthrax bacteria from these animals and grew them solely on sterile nutrients in the laboratory with no contribution from tissues or organs of the previously infected animal, and finally injected them into other uninfected animals, thereby producing anthrax in them—was the germ theory of disease proven. This occurred in 1878.

Chapter XI

Controlled scientific studies proving efficacy—or lack thereof—do not guarantee implementing or abandoning medical treatments of a given period. Although James Lind's *A Treatise on the Scurvy* showed definitively that citrus fruits treated and prevented scurvy as early as 1753, use of such fruits was not made obligatory in the Royal Navy until 1795, when Sir Gilbert Blane implemented that practice. The reason for this lapse of 40 years, in which countless sailors died of vitamin C deficiency, is unknown.

Finally, despite the publication of a detailed study in 1835 by Pierre C.A. Louis that showed blood-letting had no effect on survival of patients with several common diseases, including pneumonia and some fevers, soldiers of the Civil War were still subjected to this treatment. Perhaps its publication in French instead of English interfered with its dissemination to the United States.

Chapter XI References

1. *Medical and Surgical History of the Civil War*. Wilmington, NC: Broadfoot Publishing; Vol. I; 1990: 637. Hereafter *MSHCW*
2. *MSHCW* Vol. I; 1990: 710
3. *MSHCW* Vol. VI; 1990: 625
4. *Ibid.*, 1990: 626
5. *Ibid.*, 1990: 627
6. *Ibid.*, 1990: 629
7. Forrester RC. *Glory and Tears: Obion County, Tennessee 1860–1870*. Union City, TN: H.A. Lanzer Co.; 1966: 178
8. *Ibid.*, 213–214
9. *Ibid.*, 172
10. *MSHCW* Vol. VI; 1990: 634
11. *Ibid.*, 190: 636
12. Morton LT, Moore RJ. *A Chronology of Medicine and Related Sciences*. Brookfield, VT: Ashgate; 1997: 13
13. *Ibid.*, 41
14. *Ibid.*, 48
15. *Ibid.*, 120
16. *Ibid.*, 146

Chapter XII.
The Legacy of Civil War Surgeons

We know from the lectures heard in medical school by Walter Brice 1849 to 1851, that medicine was considered a calling that embraced an exacting code of conduct and responsibility. It is clear that surgeons serving in the War were devoted to the soldiers in their care from numerous case reports reflecting untold hours of trying to make their men comfortable and save their lives. The records also show that this war was not only about amputations, and certainly not about amputation without anesthesia. With the time-consuming ministrations using a myriad of oral medications, as well as enemas, injections, poultices, cupping, bandaging, and yes—bleeding—the expenditure of time in amputating seems, by comparison, relatively short. These surgeons observed medical standards of care developed in their era, limited by the science of their time.

Apart from exemplary service to the sick and wounded, there were important contributions by several physicians of the war. Notable among these was the systematic inquiry into how derivatives of opium work by S. Weir Mitchell.[1]

In a different vein, Union Surgeon General William Hammond tried to alleviate harm to patients from "heroic" drugs like mercury and antimony by banning their use in military service. Still others, like Jonathan Letterman and Confederate Surgeon General Samuel Preston Moore, converted dysfunctional medical departments into efficient units who removed the wounded expeditiously from the battlefield to a place of safety, pain relief and recovery, creating the framework used today to rescue wounded soldiers. Letterman organized a system by which injured men were separated (triaged) into hopelessly wounded (made comfortable) or capable of surviving their wounds; the latter progressed through his system of field dressing stations to field hospitals farther away from the battle where they were cared for. In August 1862, while Medical Director of the Army of the Potomac, Letterman reorganized ambulances and drivers so that they served in the Medical Department of the Union Army, instead of the customary Quartermaster Department. The reader is referred to the works of Bollet[2] and Rutkow[3] for the legislative details and military/medical implications of Letterman's contributions.

Surgeon John Shaw Billings, who had been a medical inspector under General Grant in the Wilderness Campaign, became the chief public health officer in the Army Medical Service and built the Library of the Office of the Surgeon General of the United States Army, which became the National Library of Medicine in 1956.[4] In 1879, Billings also began the *Index Medicus*, a critically important bibliography of medical journals, entitled then *Index Medicus: a Monthly Classified Record of the Current Medical Literature of the World*. Surgeon Joseph Janvier Woodward, chief compiler and author of the great *Medical and Surgical History of the War of the Rebellion (1861–1865)*, was one of the first to encourage the donation of specimens to the Army Medical Museum. He pioneered as a microscopist, a pathologist, and an originator of army medical laboratories as well.

Physicians who survived the 1870s, 1880s, and 1890s were alive to see the birth and development of the germ theory of disease—no more "bad air" causing infectious diseases,

Chapter XII

but living, breeding particulates that could be controlled initially in some measure by handwashing, mosquito and fly control, antisepsis with noxious substances like phenol, and wearing masks or coughing into handkerchiefs to prevent droplet-borne diseases. The most grateful patients and gratified physicians, however, would be the ones witnessing the first effective treatment of infected soldiers, using Salvarsan for syphilis in 1909, sulfa for many infections in 1935, and penicillin in 1943 for abscesses, "strep throat," gonorrhea, and pneumonia. Lest we forget the contributions of physicians serving in the Civil War, their splendid bequest to us, the monumental *Medical and Surgical History of the War of the Rebellion (1861–1865)*, authorized and published by act of Congress between 1870 and 1888, humbles us into respectful remembrance.

Chapter XII References

1. Mitchell SW. On the effect of opium and its derivative alkaloids, *Am J Med Sci* N. S. 59. 1870: 17–33
2. Bollet AJ. *Civil War Medicine Challenges and Triumphs*. Tucson, AZ: Galen Press, Ltd.; 2002: 98–101; 103–108; 455–457
3. Rutkow IM. *Bleeding Blue and Gray*. New York: Random House; 2005: 295–297
4. Bayne-Jones S. *The evolution of preventive medicine in the U.S. Army, 1607–1939*. Washington: US Government Printing Office; 1968: 106

Epilogue

Walter Brice, who had been a practicing physician in Obion County in western Tennessee since his graduation from medical school a decade before the war began, was mustered into the 9th Tennessee Infantry Regiment on May 22, 1861, at Jackson, Tennessee, as Assistant Surgeon.[1] He was appointed Surgeon by the Secretary of War, Confederate States Army, on September 26, 1861. Brice was elected regimental surgeon of the 9th Tennessee following the Battle of Shiloh (April, 1862). He passed the Medical Board examination at Chattanooga on August 23, 1862. By January of 1864 he had been appointed Regimental Surgeon of the 6th Tennessee also.[2] As such, he cared for men wounded during the Battles of Shiloh (Tennessee), Perryville (Kentucky), Murfreesboro (Tennessee), Chickamauga (Georgia), Missionary Ridge (Tennessee), Kennesaw Mountain (Georgia), Peach Tree Creek (Georgia), Atlanta (Georgia), Franklin (Tennessee), and Nashville (Tennessee).[3] The sick and wounded were his responsibility from April of 1862 until April of 1865.

The military service of Walter Brice, M.D., ended when, on April 14, 1865, General Joseph E. Johnston requested a truce for surrender from the Union Army. Consequently, on April 28, 1865, "the arms of the Ninth Tennessee Infantry were stacked around a tall tree and their battle flag was torn into fragments and distributed among its members."[4] Of 1,100 men originally in the 9th Tennessee Infantry, there remained only 46 to surrender.[4] Following the war Dr. Brice resumed his medical practice in Union City, Obion County, Tennessee. In 1870 he was elected a ruling elder of the Amalgamated Reformed Presbyterian Church in Troy, Tennessee. In 1878 he bought *The News Banner* in Union City, which he edited and managed until he sold the newspaper a decade later to his nephew James M. Brice. Dr. Brice was instrumental in founding Obion College. His obituary of November 9, 1895, notes that all his children were "students and scholars."[5]

Epilogue References

1. Cavanaugh J. *Historical Sketch of the Obion Avalanche, Company H, Ninth Tennessee Infantry, Confederate States of America*. Union City, TN: The Commercial; 1922: 172

2. Roster Of The Medical Officers Of The Army Of Tennessee. *Southern Historical Society Papers*. Richmond, VA; 1894; 22 (January-December)

3. Fleming JR. *The Ninth Tennessee Infantry: a Roster*. Shippensburg, PA: White Mane Publishing Co.; 1996: x–xv

4. Fleming JR. *The Ninth Tennessee Infantry: a Roster*. Shippensburg, PA: White Maine Publishing Co.; 1996: xv–xvi

5. Brice JM. Tribute to Dr. Walter Brice on the event of his Death, *The News Banner*, Union City, Tennessee, Nov. 9, 1895

Appendix I.

Selected References on Surgery During the Civil War

Dammann, Gordon. *Pictorial Encyclopedia of Civil War Medical Instruments and Equipment*. Missoula, Montana: Pictorial Publishing Co.; Volume I (1983); Volume II (1988); Volume III (1997)

Schaadt, Mark J. *Civil War Medicine—an Illustrated History*. Quincy, Illinois: Cedarwood Publishing, 1998

Bengtson, Bradley P. and Kuz, Julian E. *Photographic Atlas of Civil War Injuries*. Grand Rapids, Michigan: Medical Staff Press, in association with Kennesaw, GA: Kennesaw Mountain Press, Inc., 1996

Rutkow, Ira M. *The History of Surgery in the United States 1775–1900*. San Francisco: Norman Publishing; Volume I (1988); Volume II (1992)

Appendix II.

Essay Titles of 166 Students in the Class of 1851 at the University of Pennsylvania School of Medicine[1]

Dysentery/ Fevers without Rash:
Marsh miasm [malaria]
Enteric fever [associated with intestinal symptoms]
Pernicious fever
Etiology and pathology of fever
Animal heat
Enteric fever
Enteric fever
Diagnosis and treatment of enteric fever
Acute dysentery of tropical climates
Dengue as it appeared in Jacksonville in 1850
Intermittent fever
Epidemic cholera
Epidemic cholera
Enteric fever
Bilious fever [associated with liver abnormalities]
Etiology of miasmatic fevers
Enteric fever
Enteric fever
Intermittent fever
Dysentery
Remittent fever
Enteric fever
Dysentery
Bilious remittent fever
Dysentery
Enteric fever
Miasma
Diagnosis and treatment of typhus and typhoid fever
Enteric fever
Yellow fever
Intermittent fever, &c. [malaria]

Blood:
Physiology of Blood [how blood functions]
Relation of the red Blood Corpuscles [red blood cells]
Human Blood [title of Walter Brice's thesis]
Haemorrhagic Diathesis [bleeding tendency]

Miscellaneous:
Physical effects of heat and cold
Fractures [broken bones]
Dyspepsia
Animal heat
Haemorrhoids
Spinal Irritation
Etherisation [delivering anesthesia using ether]
Health versus Fashion
Phenomena of human Vision
Nausea Marina [sea sickness]
Inflammation [irritation of an organ or part of the body]
Animal Chemistry
Physiology of Digestion [how digestion occurs]
Hernia
Icterus [yellow color of skin in liver disease; jaundice]
Delirium Tremens [alcoholic delirium]
Compound Fracture [broken bone protruding through the skin]
Strictures of Urethra [scarring that causes narrowing of the urinary passage leaving the bladder]
Gun-shot Wounds
Organic Heat
The Eye and its Functions
Hepatitis [infection of the liver]
Lithiasis [kidney or bladder stones]
Empiricism [medicine founded on experience]
Acute Peritonitis [infection of the lining of the abdominal cavity]
Inguinal Hernia

Nervous System as a source of Functional and organic Disease
Sunlight
Water
Nitrogen gas
Climate of Lake Superior and its effects on Pulmonary Diseases
Vis Medicatrix Naturae [the ability of animals or plants to heal themselves]
Gastritis [irritation of the stomach lining]
Anaesthesia [anesthesia]
Concussion and Compression of Brain
The Urine
Phlegmasia Dolens [a blood clot in the deep veins of the lower leg]
Food
Inflammation
Colo-rectitis [irritation of the lower large bowel and rectum]
Diabetes
Diseases of Insanity
Hepatic Phthisis [tuberculosis of the liver]
Urea [waste product eliminated by the kidney]
Peritonitis
Inflammation
Fracture of Skull, &c.
Ascites [free fluid in the abdomen]
Gun-shot Wounds

Diseases with Rashes:
Scarlatina [scarlet fever]
Scarlatina
Scarlatina
Erysipelas
Scarlatina
Scarlatina
Idiopathic Erysipelas [severe spreading skin rash caused by streptococcus]
Variola [smallpox]

Pulmonary and Cardiac Conditions:
Consecutive Cardiac and Pulmonary Diseases
Pneumonia
Pneumonia
Pneumonia
Tuberculosis
Haemoptysis [coughing up blood]
Pneumonia
Diseases of the Heart
Pericarditis [lining around the heart]
Phthisis [tuberculosis]
Pneumonia
Mutual Dependence of the Heart and Lungs
Eccentric Hypertrophy [enlargement] of the Heart
Phthisis
Asthma
Pericarditis
Pulmonary Consumption [tuberculosis]
Endocarditis [innermost layer of the heart]
Pneumonia
Lobular Pneumonia

Therapeutics (Treatment):
Mercury
Cerated glass of antimony [wax preparation with antimony]
Opium: Its effects on the System
Ergota [ergot]
Ether
Science of Prescription
Cold as a Therapeutic Agent
Cod Liver Oil
Acidum Arseniosum [acid made of arsenic]
Physiological effects of Digitalis
Therapeutical Application of Opium
Practical Pharmacy
Cinchonia as a Tonic and Antiperiodic [quinine used as a stimulant and to suppress fever, especially that of malaria]

Obstetrics and Gynecology:
Pelvic, Podalic Version [turning the baby in a uterus to allow delivery]
Induction of Premature Labor
Irritable Uterus
Puerperal Fever ["childbed fever;" streptococcal infection after childbirth, usually fatal]

Febris Puerperal [puerperal fever]
Abortion & Sterility
Foetal Circulation
Demonstrative Midwifery
Pathologie du fetus pendant la vie intra-uterine
Secale Cornutum [ergot from rye]
Secale Cornutum as a Parturient Agent [promoting delivery]
Hysteralgia [pain in the womb]
Menstruation
Amenorrhoea [absence of menstruation]
Gonorrhea
Puerperal Fever
Inflammation of the Os and Cervix Uteri [irritation of the opening of the womb]
Physometra [inflation of the womb]
Menstruation
Puerperal Insanity
Management of Pregnancy
Merocele [a type of hernia]
Menstrual Secretion
Absorption of the Placenta
Puerperal Peritonitis [childbed fever]

Medical Education and Ethics:
Necessity of Enlightened Medical Education
Medical Reform
Study of Medicine
Medical Etiquette
Dignity of Medicine
Origin of Medicine, &c.
Medical Abstractions

Appendix II Reference

1. Horner WE. *Medical Commencement of the University of Pennsylvania held on Saturday, April 5, 1851: with a Valedictory by W. E. Horner, M.D., Professor of Anatomy.* Philadelphia: L.R. Bailey, Printer; 1851: 3–8

Appendix III.

Frequency of Rheumatic Diseases During the U.S. Civil War: Tonsillitis and Heart Disease

Tables I–VIII: The number of cases of tonsillitis in each month of the war. Month of peak incidence is shown in bold type.[1]

Table I. Tonsillitis. Army of the United States, year ending 6-30-1862

MONTH	JUL	AUG	SEP	OCT	NOV	DEC	JAN	FEB	MAR	APR	MAY	JUN
CASES	210	360	364	620	1063	1671	**1721**	1633	1369	1292	667	480
TOTAL	11,450											
DEATHS	9											
PERCENT WHO DIED	0.08%											

Table II. Tonsillitis. Army of the United States, 7-1-1862 to 6-30-1863

MONTH	JUL	AUG	SEP	OCT	NOV	DEC	JAN	FEB	MAR	APR	MAY	JUN
CASES	596	361	553	1025	1749	2529	**2702**	2390	2467	1919	1156	736
TOTAL	18,183											
DEATHS	40											
PERCENT WHO DIED	0.2%											

Table III. Tonsillitis. Army of the United States, 7-1-1863 to 6-30-1864

MONTH	JUL	AUG	SEP	OCT	NOV	DEC	JAN	FEB	MAR	APR	MAY	JUN
CASES	577	555	618	778	1178	1527	1801	2128	**2546**	2179	1030	689
TOTAL	15,606											
DEATHS	30											
PERCENT WHO DIED	0.2%											

Table IV. Tonsillitis. Army of the United States, 7-1-1864 to 6-30-1865

MONTH	JUL	AUG	SEP	OCT	NOV	DEC	JAN	FEB	MAR	APR	MAY	JUN
CASES	296	247	264	466	497	680	**884**	872	805	599	498	283
TOTAL	6,391											
DEATHS	5											
PERCENT WHO DIED		0.08%										

Table V. Tonsillitis. Army of the United States, 7-1-1865 to 6-30-1866

MONTH	JUL	AUG	SEP	OCT	NOV	DEC	JAN	FEB	MAR	APR	MAY	JUN
CASES	279	175	119	171	178	**259**	188	212	188	94	80	70
TOTAL	2,013											
DEATHS	4											
PERCENT WHO DIED		0.2%										

Table VI. Tonsillitis. Army of the United States, 7-1-1863 to 6-30-1864 (Colored Troops)

MONTH	JUL	AUG	SEP	OCT	NOV	DEC	JAN	FEB	MAR	APR	MAY	JUN
CASES	38	39	70	152	120	184	282	379	**393**	279	276	148
TOTAL	2,260											
DEATHS	3											
PERCENT WHO DIED		0.1%										

Table VII. Tonsillitis. Army of the United States, 7-1-1864 to 6-30-1865 (Colored Troops)

MONTH	JUL	AUG	SEP	OCT	NOV	DEC	JAN	FEB	MAR	APR	MAY	JUN
CASES	141	269	95	296	306	**369**	270	299	261	268	275	171
TOTAL	3,020											
DEATHS	6											
PERCENT WHO DIED		0.2%										

Appendix III.

Table VIII. Tonsillitis. Army of the United States, 7–1–1865 to 6–30–1866 (Colored Troops)

MONTH	JUL	AUG	SEP	OCT	NOV	DEC	JAN	FEB	MAR	APR	MAY	JUN
CASES	108	140	180	137	158	185	175	**190**	102	50	27	22
TOTAL	1,474											
DEATHS	3											
PERCENT WHO DIED	0.2%											

Tables IX–XVI: The number of cases of cardiac disease in each month of the war. Month of peak incidence is shown in bold type.[2]

Table IX. Heart disease. Army of the United States, year ending 6–30–1862

MONTH	JUL	AUG	SEP	OCT	NOV	DEC	JAN	FEB	MAR	APR	MAY	JUN
CASES	9	20	29	25	36	43	46	**63**	39	53	57	63
TOTAL	483											
DEATHS	78											
PERCENT WHO DIED	16%											

Table X. Heart disease. Army of the United States, 7–1–1862 to 6–30–1863

MONTH	JUL	AUG	SEP	OCT	NOV	DEC	JAN	FEB	MAR	APR	MAY	JUN
CASES	55	39	45	114	153	264	332	367	**374**	318	199	145
TOTAL	2,405											
DEATHS	405											
PERCENT WHO DIED	17%											

Table XI. Heart disease. Army of the United States, 7–1–1863 to 6–30–1864

MONTH	JUL	AUG	SEP	OCT	NOV	DEC	JAN	FEB	MAR	APR	MAY	JUN
CASES	136	174	122	127	137	135	159	155	144	**217**	152	178
TOTAL	1,836											
DEATHS	343											
PERCENT WHO DIED	19%											

Table XII. Heart disease. Army of the United States, 7–1–1864 to 6–30–1865

MONTH	JUL	AUG	SEP	OCT	NOV	DEC	JAN	FEB	MAR	APR	MAY	JUN
CASES	68	55	74	**94**	83	82	77	73	92	56	74	55
TOTAL	883											
DEATHS	160											
PERCENT WHO DIED		18%										

Table XIII. Heart disease. Army of the United States, 7–1–1865 to 6–30–1866

MONTH	JUL	AUG	SEP	OCT	NOV	DEC	JAN	FEB	MAR	APR	MAY	JUN
CASES	**94**	50	27	16	24	14	14	10	15	17	10	6
TOTAL	297											
DEATHS	52											
PERCENT WHO DIED		18%										

Table XIV. Heart disease. Army of the United States, 7–1–1863 to 6–30–1864 (Colored Troops)

MONTH	JUL	AUG	SEP	OCT	NOV	DEC	JAN	FEB	MAR	APR	MAY	JUN
CASES	3	8	5	21	26	19	21	23	**34**	27	25	25
TOTAL	237											
DEATHS	91											
PERCENT WHO DIED		38%										

Table XV. Heart disease. Army of the United States, 7–1–1864 to 6–30–1865 (Colored Troops)

MONTH	JUL	AUG	SEP	OCT	NOV	DEC	JAN	FEB	MAR	APR	MAY	JUN
CASES	28	38	43	**48**	21	31	35	30	41	21	42	49
TOTAL	427											
DEATHS	239											
PERCENT WHO DIED		56%										

Appendix III.

Table XVI. Heart disease. Army of the United States, 7–1–1865 to 6–30–1866 (Colored Troops)[2]

MONTH	JUL	AUG	SEP	OCT	NOV	DEC	JAN	FEB	MAR	APR	MAY	JUN
CASES	34	21	22	14	15	8	12	8	7	0	1	4
TOTAL	146											
DEATHS	89											
PERCENT WHO DIED		61%										

Comment: Most of these cases would have suffered abnormalities of the heart valves, a result chiefly of rheumatic fever following a sore throat or tonsillitis. There was no category for "sore throat" in the monthly reports of sickness and diseases submitted by surgeons and ultimately to the Surgeons General of Union and Confederate Armies of the Civil War. The reporting forms were arranged specifically to discern the influence of seasonal weather changes on the frequency with which many diseases occurred.

Appendix III References

1. *Medical and Surgical History of the Civil War.* Wilmington, NC: Broadfoot Publishing; Vol. I: 150–151, 300–301, 456–457, 524–525, 634–635, 668–669, 688–689, 708–709, 148–149, 298–299, 454–455, 522–523, 632–633, 666–667, 686–687, 706–707
2. *Ibid.*

Appendix IV.

Treatment of Septic Arthritis, Tracing the History of each Component, from the Text in Chapter V

1. Drainage of pus from the joint by needle and syringe, using **sterile technique**, to remove chemicals produced during infection that destroy cartilage and bone. Disinfecting the skin with chemicals (iodine or alcohol, for example) and instruments with chemicals, steam or radiation to kill bacteria and other microbes began after Robert Koch in 1878, and others, showed that living germs (present in the air, on a patient's skin, and on the hands, instruments and clothing of physicians) carry diseases.

2. Examination under a **light microscope** of a drop of the pus on a glass slide stained by Gram's method, to visualize the shape and coloration of the causative bacterium. The glass from which microscope lenses were made was of poor quality and the contour of lenses was not uniform. During the first 200 years after its development, the microscope provided a fuzzy image with colored halos around the edges and insufficient magnification to see any bacterium smaller than anthrax, until 1878. At that time Abbe, Schott and Zeiss designed and manufactured superior lenses.

3. Removal of **blood** from the patient's vein for growth in the laboratory to detect bacteria that may have "seeded" (been carried into) the joint. There are two ways that bacteria enter a joint. They may gain access through a break in the skin overlying the joint; if gunshot wounds involved a joint, fragments of germ-laden clothing were forced into a joint, further infecting it. The second route is via the normally-sterile bloodstream from an infection elsewhere in the body, e.g., an abscess. Growth of a bacterium in the bloodstream demands a search for the source of the microbe and treatment of the source. An abscess, for example, would need to be drained.

4. Administration of **antibiotics** by intravenous injection, based on the bacterium seen by microscopy. Many bacteria are eliminated by sulfa derivatives first available in 1935, but most pus-containing joints could not be successfully treated until the introduction of penicillin in 1943. Even then many failed therapy because penicillin by mouth does not enter the joint in amounts sufficient to kill bacteria. The antibiotic must be administered by intravenous injection usually several times a day for a month. Plastic tubing through which penicillin is now infused via a vein was not developed until the middle of the twentieth century. Not until 1957 was the first sterile disposable needle for a single use (Intracath® central venous catheter) designed.[1]

5. Placement of pus using sterile technique onto solid gelatin-like material (culture medium) that will nourish growth of the infecting bacterium. One of the most difficult problems in proving that one bacterium, and only one, caused one disease, and only one disease, involved separation of that bacterium from any of several other types of bacteria that might merely tag along. Initially Koch, like Pasteur, grew bacteria suspected of causing a disease in nutritious **liquid** broth that had previously been boiled to kill bacteria that might have contaminated the broth from the air. If more than one type of bacteria were inoculated into the broth, both grew mixed together in the broth and therefore could not be separated. Koch

solved the problem of isolating only one type of bacteria. He used a trick practiced by cooks to gel (solidify) their broths—he added agar to his broths. Bacteria grown on his agar-enriched growth medium in sterile shallow dishes appeared as separate solid circles (pure colonies of only one type of bacteria) that he could sample and identify under the microscope. Any contaminating bacteria could then be detected and not selected for further growth and study. Once Koch touched the appropriate colony with a sterile wand, he introduced the sample into sterile broth and grew his selected bacterium in quantity for animal studies. In 1887 Richard Julius Petri introduced the round, shallow, lidded, clear glass dishes used today to identify bacteria. They still bear his name.

6. **Identification** of the bacterium after several hours of growth (being cultured). A sterile loop (update of Koch's wand) is now used in a microbiology laboratory to transfer a bit of a bacterial colony from a Petri dish onto a slide, a piece of flat rectangular glass less than a tenth of an inch in thickness. The sample is then spread out on the slide to create a uniform thin film. When dry, the slide is placed in a series of dyes; it is then rinsed and dried. Although some bacteria can be faintly seen without being dyed, their shape and whether they are arranged singly or in pairs, chains or clumps, can be determined much more accurately with coloration. A portion of the slide is covered afterward with a smaller thinner square of glass (cover slip). Since bacteria are so small (staphylococci which cause abscesses and other serious infections are less than 1/10,000 of an inch in diameter; streptococci responsible for "strep" throats and rheumatic fever are half that size), large magnification is required to see them. The highest magnification with a light microscope is achieved by placing a drop of "immersion" oil atop the cover slip before lowering a special lens into the oil. The dyes alluded to above were developed by Hans Christian Joachim Gram in 1884. His invention permitted all bacteria to be divided into two groups. "Gram positive" bacteria turn blue and "Gram negative" ones red after dyeing. Antibiotics are generally toxic to either Gram positive or Gram negative bacteria, but not usually to both, so staining allows an initial antibiotic to be chosen, both on the basis of shape and color.

7. Further **refinement of** choice of **antibiotic** if the bacterium is not killed on culture by the antibiotic chosen initially. Once a colony grows, a sample is spread onto another Petri dish containing agar-enriched growth medium. Then small discs or strips, each containing a different antibiotic, are placed on the surface. After 24 hours, the Petri dish (plate) is examined. If a particular antibiotic is effective against the bacterium on the plate, there is a clear area around the appropriate disc, indicating the inability of the germ to grow in the neighborhood of the antibiotic. If ineffective, the bacterial colony grows right up to the periphery of the disk or strip. Accordingly, the initial antibiotic may be continued, or replaced by one that is more effective.

8. Drainage by incision in the operating room if needle drainage cannot **empty all pus** from the joint. Needle drainage in the hospital at the bedside must be done several times daily to ensure that no pus remains in the joint until the antibiotic reaches the joint in sufficient concentration and begins to kill the causative bacterium. Sometimes pus is so thick that it cannot be pulled through even a large-bore needle into a syringe, or it becomes compartmentalized, and blind needle puncture cannot locate the collection. Then the inside of the joint is visualized directly using an arthroscope, and emptied through appropriate incisions. It is critical that adequate drainage be accomplished because pus contains destructive juices (enzymes) that eat away the cartilage and bone very quickly. During the Civil War, surgeons used long cuts (several inches in length) on either side of the joint to allow egress of pus, and packed the opening with "lint" made by scraping linen with a knife blade. Of

course, knowing nothing about bacteria, surgeons did not sterilize the packing, which probably introduced additional bacteria directly into the joint.

9. Treatment of any **accompanying infection** (pneumonia, abscess, etc.). This was covered in item 3, above.

10. Institution of **physical therapy** to prevent contraction of a joint or other deformity arising from swelling or from failure of the patient to use the joint because of pain. The muscles which allow bending of the arms and legs are stronger than those that straighten them. That is why a patient who has experienced certain types of stroke has bent (contracted) wrist, elbow, shoulder, ankle, knee and hip joints on the side of the body paralyzed by the stroke. The position of comfort of a swollen painful infected joint is in the bent position, which may result in permanent bending (contracture) of the joint. Splinting or bracing the joint helps to minimize this bending. Exercises that strengthen the muscles are important to restore normal alignment of a septic joint once the infection is controlled. There were no rehabilitation physicians (physiatrists) or physical therapists, the health care professionals who evaluate and treat deformities, during the Civil War.

Comments It is easy to appreciate why joints invaded by bacteria—whether carried there by filthy clothing clinging to a bullet or borne in the bloodstream from an infection elsewhere in the body—were such a devastating development in a soldier.

Appendix IV Reference

1. Intracath® From: Becton-Dickinson web site (www.bectondickinson.com) accessed 11-10-04

Appendix V.

Prevention and Treatment of Gonorrhea during the Civil War

Freeman J. Bumstead, M.D., prepared a chapter on venereal diseases in Surgeon General William A. Hammond's book written for the U. S. Sanitary Commission, entitled *Military Medical and Surgical Essays* in July of 1864. The prophylactic practices are based on those of the Belgian Army. Bumstead advises their adoption in the Union Army. His recommendations are shown below.

    1. Every soldier who contracts venereal disease, should be required to give the name and address of the woman who infected him; and if, upon examination, she be found diseased, her removal from the neighborhood should be enforced by the military authority.

    2. Every inducement should...lead men to report themselves at the earliest possible moment after infection; and delay should be visited with appropriate penalties.

    3. No person with any venereal disease, however, slight, should be allowed to remain in quarters, but be at once transferred to the hospital.[1]

Bumstead defines three forms of sexually-transmitted disease. "There are three separate and distinct venereal diseases, viz., Gonorrhoea; the simple Chancre, or Chancroid, with its attendant bubo; and Syphilis, including the initial lesion, or true chancre, and general symptoms. The first two are local, and the last a constitutional [systemic] affection."[1] Although Bumstead discusses the treatment of all three diseases, only that of gonorrhea will appear here. Therapy of syphilis was considered in detail in Chapter IX. Mercury after Venus. Chancroid does not appear in the index of the *Medical and Surgical History of the Civil War*. The 14 complications of gonorrhea and their treatment are:

    1. The idea that gonorrhoea is dependent upon the syphilitic virus, and requires the use of mercurials, is without foundation.[1]

    2. The treatment...for most cases of gonorrhoea...[is] injections of a weak solution of some astringent, as from one to three grains of the sulphate or acetate of zinc to the ounce of water, repeated every four to six hours. [Presumably these are intraurethral.] Internally, a free purge at the outset, followed by laxatives if necessary to insure a daily evacuation from the bowels; alkaline mixtures, as solutions of the carbonates of soda or potassa, the acetate or chlorate of potassa, liquor potassae, etc., and copaiba or cubebs.[2]

    3. When the symptoms are decidedly inflammatory, they should first be subdued by rest, cathartics, and low diet, before resorting to injections. Injections are also contraindicated in cases complicated with prostatitis or cystitis.[2]

    4. Copaiva and cubebs should be given in...full doses..., but, at the same time, care should be taken not to carry them to...intolerance. Excessive action upon the bowels should be restrained by opiates or astringents, in order that their active principle may be eliminat-

ed by the kidneys and pass off in the urine. They should be suspended if they occasion uncontrollable nausea or diarrhea, a cutaneous [skin] eruption, severe pain in the kidneys, or general debility.[3]

5. Medication, both external and internal, should be continued for ten days after all discharge has ceased.[3]

6. The 'abortive treatment' of gonorrhoea is adapted only to the commencement of the disease, before acute symptoms have set in. The best formula for its administration is a weak solution of nitrate of silver...injected [into the urethra] until the discharge becomes thin and watery, (which usually takes place within twenty-four hours) and then omitted. Copaiva may be given simultaneously.[3]

7. Chordee [painful erections] may be prevented by drachm-doses [1/8 ounce] of the tincture of camphor in water, taken at bedtime.[3]

8. Commencing abscesses along the course of the urethra should be opened as soon as detected, even before fluctuation can be felt.[3]

9. Acute prostatitis may be recognized by frequent and painful micturition [urination], a throbbing pain in the perineum, and...febrile [having a fever] excitement; ...the finger introduced per anum [into the anus] detects the enlarged and sensitive gland encroaching upon the rectum. Retention of urine frequently ensues, and requires the introduction of a catheter. When the instrument reaches the prostatic portion of the urethra, it excites great pain, and meets with an obstruction, due to the swollen gland, which is readily overcome by gentle and continued pressure, the handle of the catheter at the same time being depressed. This affection may terminate in resolution or in suppuration [formation of pus]. The latter is announced by repeated chills; and, if the abscess points toward the rectum, fluctuation may be detected by the finger introduced per anum; more frequently, however, the matter tends to escape by the urethra.[4]

10. Acute prostatitis is to be treated at its commencement by absolute rest, cups followed by poultices to the perineum, warm baths, and laxatives or enemata. The bladder should be evacuated, when necessary, with the catheter. If suppuration ensues, the abscess should be opened at an early period in whichever direction it tends to point, either with a knife through the rectum, or with the point of a catheter through the urethra.[4]

11. Gonorrhoeal cystitis is commonly limited to the neck of the bladder. Its symptoms are an urgent and frequent desire to empty the bladder; sharp pain attending the flow of the last drops of urine; the admixture of pus or blood with this fluid; tenderness of the hypogastric [stomach] region; pain radiating to the groins, perineum, anus, and along the course of the urethra. There is usually less...[fever] than in acute prostatitis.[5]

12. Gonorrhoeal cystitis is...treated by rest, warm baths, cups, and poultices to the hypogastria, and internally by saline laxatives, the carbonates of soda and potassa, the acetate or chlorate of potassa, liquor potassae, mucilage, flaxseed tea, and copaiba.[5]

13. Gonorrhoeal epididymitis (swelled testicle) is best treated by the horizontal posture; support of the scrotal organs; and emetico-cathartic, as a solution of Epsom salts and tartarized antimony, given in sufficient doses to act freely upon the bowels and maintain slight nausea; the application of leeches or cups just below the external abdominal ring, or bleeding from the scrotal veins—(the patient in a standing posture, and the scrotum compressed at its neck, either with the hand or a fillet [a cord for putting traction on the scrotum], and bathed with hot water until its veins are well distended;) and hot poultices, either of

flaxseed or tobacco leaves, to the affected part. Evacuate any collection of fluid in the tunica vaginalis [inner lining of the testicle]; and, even in the absence of any marked degree of hydrocele [a collection of fluid in the testicle], Velpeau's treatment by means of multiple punctures with a lancet is worthy of a trial. When the acute symptoms have subsided, employ a more tonic regimen and strap the affected testicle. Mild urethral injections are not contraindicated by the occurrence of swelled testicle.[5]

14. Gonorrhoeal ophthalmic [eye infection] requires the strictest attention to cleanliness, the frequent use of an astringent collyrium [eyewash], freedom of the bowels, and, in most cases, tonics or stimulants. The eyes should be bathed every fifteen minutes with a solution of a drachm of alum to a pint of tepid water, or a decoction of poppy heads. The surgeon, at his daily visit, after thoroughly cleansing the mucous membrane of its purulent secretion and the adherent masses of coagulum, should snip the chemosed [swollen conjunctiva around the cornea] portions of the ocular conjunctiva with scissors, and, after the bleeding has ceased, pencil the whole affected surface either with the solid crayon of nitrate of silver, or with a strong solution of the same salt, …washing off the residue with tepid water as soon as the surface has become whitened. In addition, a solution of five grains of nitrate of silver to the ounce of water may be dropped in the eye three or four times a day by the attendant. An active purge at the outset of treatment is desirable, and a daily evacuation of the bowels should be secured. The great danger to vision is from ulceration and slough of the cornea, a tissue of low vitality, and a disastrous termination of the disease is favored by a low condition of the general system; hence all depressing agents, as venesection [therapeutic bleeding], mercurials, tartarized antimony, abstinence from food, etc., are to be avoided, and a nourishing diet, porter, ale, quinine, and other tonics, to be enjoined. If ulceration of the cornea occurs, its progress may perhaps be arrested by lightly touching the surface with a pointed crayon of nitrate of silver; and the pupil should be constantly dilated with atropine or belladonna. Poultices of every kind are to be strictly prohibited, and the eye left uncovered. The discharge is highly contagious, and the utmost caution should be used to prevent its coming in contact with a sound eye.[6] [Solution of silver nitrate is still placed on the eyeballs of newborns to prevent eye infection while the child is traversing the birth canal, in case the mother has gonorrhea.]

Comment: This Appendix is included to show the astute observational skills of some surgeons of the time—especially important since diagnostic instruments were either not yet developed or primitive by today's standards. It also demonstrates that some physicians of the period followed protocols, and were not just using individual preferences, to treat certain diseases. Finally the reader is made aware of the horrific complications of gonorrhea in the pre-penicillin era. Penicillin was not even widely available in World War II until 1944.

Appendix V References

1. Bumstead FJ. Venereal Diseases. In: *Military Medical and Surgical Essays prepared for the United States Sanitary Commission*. ed. Hammond WA. Philadelphia: J.B. Lippincott and Co.; 1864: 532
2. *Ibid.*, 533
3. *Ibid.*, 533–534
4. *Ibid.*, 534–535
5. *Ibid.*, 535–536
6. *Ibid.*, 537–538

Appendix VI.

Preparations of Mercury Still in Use *

Mercurochrome (Merbromin). Used as an antiseptic; in microscopy to stain cytoplasm of cells, and in bright–field and fluorescence microscopy.

Mercuric chloride (corrosive sublimate, mercury bichloride, mercury perchloride, corrosive mercury perchloride, corrosive mercury chloride), $HgCl_2$. A topical antiseptic and disinfectant for "inanimate objects."

Mercuric iodide, red (mercury biniodide, mercury deutiodide), HgI_2. Antiseptic and disinfectant for inanimate objects.

Mercuric oxide, red (red precipitate). "The red precipitate of HgO; ...used externally as an antiseptic in chronic skin diseases and fungus infections."

Mercuric oxide, yellow (yellow precipitate). "The yellow precipitate of HgO; used externally as antiseptic and in the treatment of inflammatory conditions of the eyelids and the conjuntivae."

Mercuric salicylate (mercury subsalicylate). "A powder used externally in the treatment of parasitic and fungus skin diseases."

Mercurous chloride (calomel), HgCl.

Ammoniated mercury (ammoniated mercuric chloride, white mercuric precipitate), $HgNH_2Cl$. "Used in ointment for the treatment of skin diseases."

Comment: As late as 1975, mercury was still used as a diuretic. It was the only such medication during the thirty years before that!

* From *Stedman's Medical Dictionary*, 26th ed. Baltimore: Williams & Wilkins; 1995: 1091

Appendix VII.

Surgeries Performed with Ether or Chloroform July 19, 1847, to February 26, 1848, by Faculty of University of Pennsylvania School of Medicine and Jefferson Medical College

Operations performed using ether by University of Pennsylvania faculty:
1. Repaired anal fissure
2. Amputation of leg
3. Extirpation of fungus of eyeball
4. Repaired anal fissure
5. Necrosis (bone death) of tibia [shin]
6. Extirpation of breast cancer
7. Repaired perineal [between the scrotum and anus or between the vulva and the anus] fistula
8. Necrosis of femur [bone death, thigh]
9. Removal of scalp cyst
10. Repaired anal fistula

Operations performed using chloroform by University of Pennsylvania faculty:
11. Repaired perineal fistula
12. Repaired urethral stricture
13. Repaired urethral stricture

Operations performed using ether at the Clinic of the Jefferson Medical College:
1. Resected [amputation] stump
2. Removed fungous testis
3. Removed wens [cysts] of scalp
4. Extirpated fungus of eyeball
5. Amputated thigh
6. Removed tumor of shoulder
7. Excised breast cancer
8. Removed tumour of scalp
9. Operated anal fistula
10. Amputated finger
11. Operated burn deformity
12. Removed tumour of neck
13. Operated anal fistula
14. Removed tumour of scalp
15. Removed tumour of thigh
16. Extracted cartilage of knee joint
17. Removed inverted toenail
18. Removed tumour of neck
19. Removed tumour of jaw
20. Operated anal fistula
21. Operated ectropium [rolled out eyelid]

22. Removed lupus [tuberculosis] tumour
23. Removed inverted toenail
24. Removed chancroid [venereal soft chancre] tumour
25. Operated phimosis [narrowing requiring circumcision]
26. Operated anal fistula
27. Resected humerus [upper arm]
28. Removed breast cancer
29. Operated anal fistula
30. Excised breast cancer
31. Removed lupus tumour
32. Removed lupus of eye
33. Excised tumour zygoma [cheekbone]

Operations performed using chloroform by Jefferson faculty:
34. Removed upper jaw for tumour
35. Removed testicle
36. Removed tumour of breast
37. Removed tumour of shoulder
38. Operated hemorrhoids
39. Removed tumour of shoulder
40. Operated eyelid
41. Amputated leg
42. Removed tumour of head
43. Removed tumour of face
44. Removed wens from scalp[1]

Appendix VII Reference

1. *Trans AMA,* Vol. I. 1848: 176; 220–221

Appendix VIII.
History of Smallpox Prophylaxis

Sometimes there is an ancient body of work providing evidence that prophylaxis against a disease is effective. Such is the case with smallpox. Bayne-Jones reviews its fascinating history. Cotton Mather (1663–1728), clergyman, "stimulated Zabdiel Boylston to immunize against smallpox by inoculation (variolation) in Boston in 1721. This was the first positive achievement in preventive medicine in the Colonies."[1] Not only that, but Mather (and Boylston) kept records of who was vaccinated. Mather "reported to the Royal society, during the severe Boston epidemic of [smallpox in] 1721, that more than one in six of all who took the disease in the natural fashion died; but that out of three hundred inoculated, only about one in sixty died."[2]

Bayne-Jones reports:

> Inoculation against smallpox (the insertion into a normal individual, by scarification or puncture, of material from a fresh lesion of smallpox, with the intention to produce a mild attack of the disease) was an ancient practice of the Chinese and had been utilized in Africa since an uncertain time long past. It came to notice in England about 1700, and in 1714 and 1716, the royal Society of London published in its 'Philosophical Transactions' favorable accounts by Emanuel Timoni, of Constantinople, and Jacobus Pylarini, of Venice. In April 1721, the first inoculation in England was performed on the daughter of lady Mary Wortly Montagu. Thereafter having been taken up by royalty and found relatively safe and a safeguard, inoculation became widely practiced in England and in Europe. It was applied in the British Army with increasing frequency before the start of the American Revolutionary War.[3]
>
> By the time of the [American] Revolution, inoculation was practiced on general preventive grounds in the Colonies as it was in England....[4]

Effecting immunity by using material from the scabs of a smallpox victim was the only method known until Edward Jenner discovered and published a safer way—with scabs of those who had contracted a related but different disease, cowpox. His masterful account of cowpox and its ability to prevent the dreaded smallpox, in *The Vaccine Inquirer* of 1822, reads thus:

> The deviation of man from the state in which he was originally placed by nature seems to have proved to him a prolific source of diseases... What makes the cow pox so extremely singular, is, that the person who has been thus infected, is for ever after secure from the infection of the small pox; — neither exposure to...[smallpox], nor the insertion of...matter [from smallpox sores] into the skin, producing this distemper. [When cowpox infects cows it spreads] from the cows to the dairymaids...[and] spreads through the farm until most of the cattle and...[domestic workers develop the disease]. It

appears on the nipples of the cows in the form of irregular pustules....
...Inflamed spots now begin to appear on different parts of the hands of the domestics employed in milking, and sometimes on the wrists. [The spots take on] a circular form, with their edges more elevated than their center, and of a colour distantly approaching to blue.... [Tumors then appear in each armpit], the pulse is quickened, and shiverings, succeeded by heat, with general lassitude, and pains about the loins and limbs, with vomiting come on. The head is painful, and the patient is now then affected with delirium...from day 1 to 3 or 4, leaving ulcerated sores about the hands...and heal slowly.[5]

Although Jenner's patients with cowpox became ill, none of them died. In the same issue of *The Vaccine Inquirer* it is stated that in the United States vaccination with cowpox began in Maryland in 1801. Material from a sore of a patient ill with cowpox was shipped from London (from Dr. Jenner) to Dr. James Smith in Baltimore County. Smith describes that the material "was put up for its more certain preservation, in three different ways: some on the blade of a lancette [small blade with a handle], some between small plates of glass; and some on thread which was thoroughly charged with it; and the whole was confined in a vial well corked and sealed." Once people were vaccinated, most were tested by injecting them with smallpox, and all developed a weeping elevated sore that formed a scab. There were either no other symptoms or at most a slight fever. None came down with smallpox.[6] Vaccination was performed also in Philadelphia in 1801, using matter obtained from Thomas Jefferson, who acquired it from Dr. Benjamin Waterhouse of Cambridge, who received it from Jenner. Jefferson inoculated 70 or 80 of his family and neighbors after 1800.[6] Dr. James Smith wrote an article, *Observations on Cow Pox*, in the same issue of the journal, recommending " vaccine inoculation to all who never having had the small pox, justly regard their own safety or that of their children and friends."[7] He even wrote a letter to the 15th Congress of the U.S. in 1812 advocating vaccination of all the population:

The natural small pox is now taking a wide range through this and the adjacent states, and many thousand lives may be reasonably expected a sacrifice to it during this spring and the ensuing summer, unless those who are liable to take it, can be generally persuaded to adopt the use of the kine-pock [another term for cow pox]—a remedy which, however inscrutable may be its operation..., has power to rescue the human race from the most destructive pestilence which has ever afflicted them.[8]

Smith even enclosed "some genuine vaccine matter" with his letter. He also offered to examine the scab (crust) from anyone inoculated with cowpox to be certain he received cowpox and not a spurious inoculation. Smith gave specific instructions on how to send the scab:

As soon as the scabs or crusts become loose they should be taken off and wrapped in a little fine lint or cotton; they may then be folded up in a small piece of clean white paper, on which must be written the name, age, and place of residence, of the person or persons from whom they were taken; and also the time when they came off. In all cases thus submitted, where the vaccination has been effectual, a certificate signed by the subscriber will be given,

Appendix VIII

declaring that the person who has been the subject of it will never thereafter be liable to take the small pox; and if any vaccination may be found to have been spurious, imperfect, or ineffectual, the necessary precautions to be taken, will be particularly and promptly given in a *letter of advice* [italics in original].[9]

Studies published in 1822 documented the efficacy of universal vaccination in Europe. In the 12 years preceding vaccination in Denmark, there were 5,500 deaths from smallpox in Copenhagen alone. In 1805 not one death occurred in the entire country. In 1800 laws were enacted that "no person should be received at confirmation, admitted to any school, bound apprentice to any trade, or married, who had not been vaccinated, unless they had undergone the small pox."[10] In Prussia in 1817 deaths from smallpox were reduced from 1 in 7 to 1 in 104.[11] Of interest, in France annual prizes were awarded to doctors who vaccinated the largest number of people.[11]

As discussed in Chapter XI, there were several reasons why soldiers developed smallpox during the Civil War, despite the solid evidence that prophylaxis was effective.

Appendix VIII References

1. Bayne-Jones S. *The evolution of preventive medicine in the U.S. Army, 1607–1939*. Washington: U.S. Government Printing Office; 1968: 16
2. *Ibid.*, 19
3. *Ibid.*, 17
4. *Ibid.*, 21
5. Jenner E. An inquiry into the causes and effects of the varioloe vaccinoe, a disease discovered in some of the western counties of England—particularly Gloucestershire, and known by the name of the cowpox, London 1798. In: *The Vaccine Inquirer*, Vol. I. Baltimore: John D. Toy; 1822: 1–15
6. *The Vaccine Inquirer*, Vol. I. Baltimore: John D. Toy; 1822: 16–23
7. *Ibid.*, 35–37
8. Smith J. *The Vaccine Inquirer*, Vol. I. Baltimore: John D. Toy; 1822: 41
9. *Ibid.*, 42–43
10. *The Vaccine Inquirer*, Vol. I. Baltimore: John D. Toy; 1822: 95
11. *The Vaccine Inquirer*, Vol. I. Baltimore: John D. Toy; 1822: 96

Appendix IX.

Inflammation

Dunglison's Definition, 1846:[1]

In, "within" and *flamma*, "flame or fire." An irritation in a part of the body occasioned by some stimulus; —owing to which the blood flows into the capillary vessels in greater abundance than natural, and those vessels become over-dilated and enfeebled; whence result pain, redness, heat, tension, and swelling; symptoms which appear in greater or less severity, according to the structure, vital properties, and functions of the part affected, and its connexion [sic] with other parts, as well as according to the constitution of the individual. The inflammations of the cellular and serous membranes greatly agree; —and those of the mucus and skin; the former being more active, and constituting the *phlegmonous* variety; —the latter, the erythematic, or *erysipelatous*. Inflammation may end by resolution, suppuration, gangrene, adhesion, effusion, or induration. Each of the inflammations of internal organs has received a name according to the organ affected; —as, *gastritis, cephalitis, enteritis, hepatitis*, &c.

Examination of the blood drawn, always exhibits an increase of the fibrinous [fibrin is a protein in the blood] element —the average proportion of which, in healthy blood, is 3 in the thousand. In inflammation, it at times rises as high as 10. In fevers unaccompanied with inflammation, the proportion is natural or below the average; but whenever inflammation supervenes, it immediately rises.

External inflammation is easily detected by the characters already mentioned: —internal, by disturbance of function and pain upon pressure, but the last sign is often not available. Both forms require the removal of all irritation, and the reduction of vascular excitement and nervous irritability; hence, blood-letting—local and general—sedatives, refrigerants, and counter-irritants become valuable remedies in almost all cases of inflammation.

Stedman's definition of inflammation, 1995:[2]

A fundamental pathologic process consisting of a dynamic complex of cytologic and chemical reactions that occur in the affected blood vessels and adjacent tissues in response to an injury or abnormal stimulation caused by a physical, chemical, or biologic agent, including: 1) the local reactions and resulting morphologic changes, 2) the destruction or removal of the injurious material, 3) the responses that lead to repair and healing. The so-called 'cardinal signs' of…[inflammation] are: *rubor*, redness; *calor*, heat (or warmth); *tumor*, swelling; and *dolor*, pain; a fifth sign, *functio laesa*, inhibited or lost function, is sometimes added. All of the signs may be observed in certain instances, but no one of them is necessarily always present.

Comment: It is remarkable that much of the language is the same in these two definitions written 150 years apart.

Appendix IX References

1. Dunglison R. *A Dictionary of Medical Science*. Philadelphia: Lea and Blanchard; 1846: 406
2. *Stedman's Medical Dictionary*, 26th ed., Baltimore: Williams & Wilkins; 1995: 869

Appendix X.

Classification of Medications and Pertinent Passages from *Carson's Materia Medica of 1851*[1]

I. SUBSTANCES WHICH ACT ON THE SOLIDS AND FLUIDS OF THE BODY.

Stimulants	Permanent	Astringents Tonics	
	Diffusible	Arterial Cerebro-nervous	Nervous Cerebral Excito-motor
Sedatives	Arterial Nervous		
Alteratives			
Affecting functions	Emetics Cathartics Diuretics Diaphoretics Expectorants Emmenagogues Sialogogues Errhines		
Affecting organization	Epispastics Rubefacients Escharotics		
Operating mechanically	Demulcents Emollients Diluents		

II. SUBSTANCES WHICH ACT ON FOREIGN MATTER IN THE BODY.

Antacids
Anthelmintics

Astringents.

"Astringents are substances which, when applied to the tissues of the living body, cause them to contract, and, as consequence, increase their firmness and density." Examples are QUERCUS TINCTORIA (*Black Oak Bark*), used for poultices; and ALUMEN, U.S. (*Alum; Sulphate of Alumina and Potassa*), formed from "alum ore," and used to control bleeding.

Tonics.

"These medicines...produce a gentle and persistent exaltation of the vital movements, and thereby give strength and vigor to the... system." An example of a "bitter tonic" is CINCHONA (*Peruvian Bark*), bark of [several] species of *Cinchona* from the western coast of South America. A "mineral tonic" is exemplified by FERRUM (*Iron*); it is used in "cases of debility,...where there is an impoverished state of the blood...attendant upon anaemia."

Arterial stimulants.

"They differ from tonics in acting rapidly and forcibly....They are employed in cases of debility, with great depression of the vital powers, and where there is prostration, and tendency to collapse." Examples are SPIRITUS AMMONIAE (*Spirit of Ammonia*) and OLEUM TEREBINTHINAE (*Oil of Turpentine*).

Nervous stimulants.

"These...[exert]...a stimulating impression upon the nervous system and...the brain...." One such is COFFEA (*Coffee*), from seeds of *Coffea arabica*, which contain *caffein*.

Cerebral stimulants.

"These are substances which...have a...special direction to the brain.... Although the primary effect is stimulating, it is soon followed by depression and subsidence of the vital actions.... Sleep is the most prominent effect induced by them; hence they have been termed *Narcotics*, *Soporifics*, [and] *Hypnotics;* and, as they relieve pain, they have also been called *Anodynes*." One example is MORPHIA, derived from opium, which exists as *Narcotina* or *Codeia*. Another is BELLADONNA (*Belladonna*), from leaves of *Atropa belladonna* (*Deadly nightshade*), which contain *Atropia*. It dilates the pupil of the eye. Two act as anesthetics: AETHER (*Ether*), or *Aether Sulphuricus;* and CHLOROFORMUM (*Chloroform*).

Excito-motor stimulants.

"They are used either to arouse muscular structure into action..., or to gently bring about lost motor power in muscles." Exemplified by NUX VOMICA (*Nux vomica*), from seeds of the *Strychnos nux vomica*. They contain *Strychnia*.

Arterial sedatives.

"Arterial Sedatives...depress the circulation; diminish the force and frequency of the

heart's action; lower the pulse; [and] diminish the number...[of breaths per minute]...."
Best known are TARTAR EMETIC (*Antimonium Tartarizatum*), POTASSAE NITRAS (*Nitrate of Potassa, Nitre, Saltpeter*) and ACIDUM ACETICUM (*Acetic Acid, Vinegar*).

Nervous sedatives.

"Such substances...produce a marked diminution of nervous power, and...at the same time...reduce the force of the circulation...." Three prominent examples are DIGITALIS (*Foxglove*), from leaves of *Digitalis purpurea, Foxglove*, which contain *Digitalin*; TABACUM (*Tobacco*), from leaves of the *Nicotiana tabacum*, that contain *Nicotina*; and ACONITUM, from leaves or root of *Aconitum napellus* (*Wolfsbane; Monkshood*), which contain *Aconitina*. This substance is "a powerful irritant to the skin when locally applied. A powerful sedative, with...[an] anodyne property...[when given by mouth]."

Alteratives.

"Alterative medicines...produce...in the organs and tissues...healthy action...to take the place of diseased action. Under proper control, they act slowly, but safely; no appreciable action [such as vomiting or sweating or purging] is to be discovered; but, with the removal of diseased structural conditions, disordered functions assume their natural state." These agents include mercury, iodine, and arsenic.

Emetics.

These "produce a discharge of the contents of the stomach through...the mouth...[by] *vomiting*." The stomach is evacuated "in cases of ingestion of poisons; to unload...the pancreas, liver, lungs, and bowels; *to reduce arterial circulation, and relax the system*, [acting as an]...*antiphlogistic* [against irritation or inflammation]." Agents in this category are IPECACUANHA (*Ipecacuanha*), the source of which is *Cephoelis ipecacuanha, Richardsonia scabra*, or *Psychotria emetica*; ANTIMONII ET POTASSAE TARTRAS (*Tartar Emetic*), employed in fevers and hepatitis; and zinc or copper sulphate.

Cathartics.

These agents are used *to "unload the bowels"* of the "evils of confined bowels," or to deplete or relieve the circulation in febrile (feverish) "affections." Examples are OLEUM RICINI (*Castor Oil*), from seeds of *Ricinus communis*; JALAPA (*Jalap*), from root of *Ipomoea Jalapa* of Mexico; PODOPHYLLUM (*Mayapple*), from root of *Podophyllum peltatum*; COLOCYNTHIS (*Colocynth*), from fruit of *Citrullus colocynthis*; and HYDRARGYRI CHLORIDUM MITE (*Calomel*).

Enemata (**Enemas**).

Used to "facilitate the action of Cathartic Medicines, or simply to open the bowels," using warm water, flaxseed tea, elm bark, barley water, Senna tea, castor oil, or *Oil of Turpentine*.

Diuretics.

"These are medicines which occasion increased action of the kidneys, and promote the...secretion" of urine. One indication is *"to evacuate fluid"* in dropsies (fluid accumulation in heart failure and in kidney or liver disease). Examples are SCILLA (*Squill*) from *Scilla maritima;* COLCHICHI RADIX or COLCHICI SEMEN (*Colchicum Seed* or *Colchicum Root*); DIGITALIS (*Foxglove*); TEREBINTHINA (*Turpentine*), from juice of *Pinus palustris* and other pines trees; COPAIBA (*Copaifera*); and CANTHARIS (*Cantharides,* Spanish Flies).

Diaphoretics.

These "medicines...produce or facilitate the discharge from the *skin: Citrullus colocynthis*; and HYDRARGYRI CHLORIDUM MITE. When moderate, ...perspiration; when profuse, sweat." Examples are IPECACUANHA, POTASSAE CITRAS (*Citrate of Potassa*), and SASSAFRAS RADICIS CORTEX (*Bark of Sassafras Root*).

Expectorants.

These "facilitate expectoration, or the discharge of matters from the lungs, which, if retained, would give rise to difficulty of breathing...." Some of these are *Tartar Emetic; Ipecacuanha,* SCILLA (*Squill*); and BENZOINUM (*Benzoin*), juice of *Styrax benzoin*.

Emmanagogues.

These are "substances which promote the functional action of the uterus, and which provoke and maintain the periodical occurrence of the menstrual secretion." Medicines in this class include GUAIACA RESINA (*Guaiac*), HELLOBORUS NIGER (*Black Hellebore*), and SABINA (*Savin*) from the tops of *Juniperus sabina*.

Sialogogues.

Substances that produce salivary discharge are designated by this term. One such is PYRETHRUM, U.S. (*Pellitory*). The root of the *Anacylus pyrethrum*. Mercury is excluded, since it works throughout the system, and not just locally, to increase saliva.

Errhines.

Medicines used to promote nasal secretion. No examples are given.

Epispastics.

"Substances which, by their action upon the skin, produce a blister. Sometimes the terms *Blisters* and *Vesicatories* are used to designate them." They relieve inflammation or congestion. One such is CANTHARIS (*Spanish Flies; Cantharis vesicatoria*). Native to Spain and Italy, flies are ground into a powder. CANTHARIS VITTATA (*Potato Flies*) are also used.

Appendix X

Rubefacients.

Articles "which redden the skin in consequence of the irritation and inflammation they produce...." Members of this group are SINAPIS (*Mustard*), from seeds of *Sinapis nigra* and *Sinapis alba*; CAPSICUM (*Cayenne Pepper*); OLEUM TEREBINTHINAE (*Oil of Turpentine*); LIQUOR AMMONIAE (*Solution of Ammonia*); PIX BURGUNDICA (*Burgundy Pitch*); PIX CANADENSIS (*Canada Pitch*); and *Hemlock Pitch*.

Escharotics.

"Substances which destroy vitality in the part to which applied, producing disorganization, and a slough." "They are used to remove diseased growths," to "alter the action in diseased parts," and "to open abscesses...." Examples are POTASSA (*Potassa, Caustic Potassa,* "energetic" caustic; ACIDUM ARSENICUM (*Arsenious Acid*); ARGENTI NITRAS FUSUS (*Fused Nitrate of Silver, Lunar Caustic*); and HYDRARGYRI CHLORIDUM CORROSIVUM (*Corrosive Chloride of Mercury*).

Demulcents.

"These are bland substances, readily dissolved by water, and which produce a calming, soothing effect upon irritated or inflamed surfaces." Three of these are ACACIA (*Gum Arabic*), the juice of *Acacia vera*, "soothing" and used in cough mixtures; LINUM (*Flaxseed*), from seeds of *Linum usitatissimum*, the common *Flax*; GLYCYRRHIZA (*Liquorice Root*), from *Glycyrrhiza glabra*; and TAPIOCA (*Tapioca*), from the root of *Janipha manihot*.

Emollients.

"Bland and unirritating substances, which...retain heat and moisture," they "are adapted for the formation of Poultices and Cataplasms, which are employed to soften [and]...relax" the skin.

Diluents.

Water is the main liquid for diluting the concentration of medicines; the demulcents also are in this group when used to dilute the contents of the stomach and bowels.

Antacids.

"These substances neutralize the injurious properties of acids by combining with them in the stomach and bowels." They are...alkalies...and, by combination with acids, neutral salts are formed, which may be absorbed and eliminated by the kidneys.... Exemplified by LIQUOR POTASSAE (*Solution of Potassa*); SODAE CARBONAS (*Carbonate of Soda*); and SODAE BICARBONAS (*Bicarbonate of Soda*).

Anthelmintics.

"These medicines aid or cause the expulsion of worms from the ...[intestines,] by debilitating them, and enabling purgatives to remove them; or by destroying their vitality." Examples are SPIGELIA (*Pinkroot, Starblom, Carolina Pink*), from root of *Spigelia mari-*

landica; CHENOPODIUM (*Wormseed, Jerusalem Oak*), from fruit of *Chenopodium anthelminticum*; and AZEDARACH, U.S. (*Azedarach*), from the bark of the root of *Melia Azedarach*.

Comment: This classification is included so the reader may appreciate that medical school faculty who trained doctors destined to serve in the Civil War were systematic in their approach to medicines and tried to comprehend how drugs work. It also provides examples of medicines in each category, as well as the ingredients of many substances that will be encountered by a student of Civil War medicine.

Appendix X Reference

1. Dorwart BB. *Carson's Materia Medica of 1851: An Annotation*. Bala Cynwyd, PA: WVD Press; 2003: 11–76

* Carson's fonts have been preserved throughout the document.

Appendix XI.

Using the Broadfoot Index of 1991[1] to Access the Original Six-volumes of *The Medical and Surgical History of the War of the Rebellion (1861–1865)*[2]

Context: *The Medical and Surgical History of the War of the Rebellion (1861–1865)* [*MSHWR*] did not have an index until all of its six volumes were computer-scanned in their entirety and indexed by Broadfoot Publishing in 1991. Except for the title, *The Medical and Surgical History of the Civil War*, this reprint in 12 volumes, not including the Index, is identical to the original work. This is obviously a great boon to researchers of Civil War medicine, but it requires detailed adherence to the following instructions to mesh these two works effectively. Note: Although the Broadfoot index has three volumes, only Vol. II and Vol. III house the *medical index*. (Vol. I, "Entries by State and Unit," contains names of soldiers, and no medical data.)

The following steps are suggested:

Set up the original *MSHWR* volumes *in this order*, being certain of exact *title* and whether numbers are *Roman* or *Arabic* on the binding of *each* of the *six* volumes:

"Medical Vol. & Appendix" (1875), Part 1, Vol. 1

"Medical History" (1879), Part 2, Vol. 1

"Medical History" (1888), Part 3, Vol. 1

"Part First Surgical Volume" (1875)

"Surgical History" (1877), Part 2, Vol. 2

"Surgical History" (1883), Part III, Vol. II

Select item you wish to find in Broadfoot index. It will have a Roman numeral and an Arabic page number. E.g., " scurvy" is listed II, 55–56; IV, 495–496.

Using this table, find your item in its respective volume of *MSHWR*:

Broadfoot I = "Medical Vol. & Appendix," Part 1, Vol. 1, pp. 1 through 726, but not the Appendix to Part 1.

Broadfoot II = "Medical Vol. & Appendix," Part 1, Vol. 1, pp. 1 through 353, which is Appendix to Part 1.

Broadfoot III = "Medical History," Part 2, Vol. 1, pp. 1 through 482.

Broadfoot IV = "Medical History," Part 2, Vol. 1, pp. 483–842

Broadfoot V = "Medical History," Part 3, Vol. 1, pp. 1 through 480.

Broadfoot VI = "Medical History," Part 3, Vol. 1, pp. 481 through 966.

Broadfoot VII = "Part First Surgical Volume," pp. 1 through 266. Note that you have to wade through *Prefatory, Introduction, Chronological Summary of Engagements and Battles*, which comprise virtually the first half of this volume, before arriving at page 1!

Broadfoot VIII = "Part First Surgical Volume," pp. 267 through 650.

Broadfoot IX = "Surgical History," Part 2, Vol. 2, pp. 1 through 472.

Broadfoot X = "Surgical History," Part 2, Vol. 2, pp. 473 through 1024.

Broadfoot XI = Surgical History, Part III, Vol. II, pp. 1 through 426.

Broadfoot XII = Part III, Vol. II, pp. 427 through 986.

Example: " Scurvy" in Broadfoot index is II, 55–56; and also IV, 495–496. The first entry will be in *MSHWR* "Medical Vol. & Appendix," Part 1, Vol. 1, which is the Appendix to Part 1, on pp. 55–56. The second entry will be in "Medical History," Part 2, Vol. 1, pp. 495–496.

Prepared by Bonnie Brice Dorwart, M.D., Fellow of the College of Physicians of Philadelphia, with the assistance of Richard Fraser, Medical Librarian at that institution.

Appendix XI References

1. *Medical and Surgical History of the Civil War.* Wilmington, NC, Broadfoot Publishing; 1991
2. *Medical and Surgical History of the War of the Rebellion (1861–1865).* Washington, D.C., Government Printing Office; 1875–1888

Appendix XII.

Excerpts from Lectures Heard by Walter Brice, M.D., at the University of Pennsylvania School of Medicine 1849–1851, and the Professors who Gave Them

Subjects of Brice's lectures and professors for the 1849–1850 session were:

Theory and Practice of Medicine	Nathaniel Chapman
Anatomy	William E. Horner
Materia Medica and Pharmacy	George Bacon Wood
Chemistry	James B. Rogers
Surgery	William Gibson
Obstetrics and the Diseases of Women and Children	Hugh L. Hodge
Institutes of Medicine	Samuel Jackson[1]

Professors during the 1850–1851 session were:

Theory and Practice of Medicine	George Bacon Wood
Anatomy	William E. Horner
Materia Medica and Pharmacy	Joseph Carson
Chemistry	James B. Rogers
Surgery	William Gibson
Obstetrics and the Diseases of Women and Children	Hugh L. Hodge
Institutes of Medicine	Samuel Jackson[2]

Portraits of each appear in Figures 1–8. *All are from the Library of the College of Physicians of Philadelphia.*

As noted in Chapter II, these lectures survive because medical students paid for the publication of ones they felt should be published. Correspondence arranging publication of one shows Walter Brice on the committee. The letter is as follows, with the original case lettering:

University of Pennsylvania, Oct. 9th, 1850

Professor Jackson:

Dear Sir—At a meeting of the Medical Class of the University of Pennsylvania, the undersigned were appointed a Committee to request for publication a copy of your truly able and eloquent Introductory Address, delivered October 9th, 1850.

Hoping that you will comply with their request, we are, sir, with sentiments of high regard,

> Very respectfully yours,
> JOHN H. DECHERD, Tennessee,
> ANDREW R. BARBEE, Jr., Virginia,
> Walter Brice, South Carolina,
> JAMES H. TURNER, Virginia,
> JAMES P. BURKE, Tennessee,
> Committee.

Samuel Jackson, M.D., Professor of the Institutes of Medicine, replied:

> Phila., Oct. 9th, 1850.
>
> To Messrs. John H. Decherd, Tennessee, Andrew R. Barbee, Jr., Virginia, Walter Brice, South Carolina, James H. Turner, Virginia, James P. Burke, Tennessee, Committee.
>
> GENTLEMEN—Your note of this date, requesting a copy of my Introductory Address, was receive [sic] this evening.
>
> I cannot refuse to comply with the wishes of the highly respectable body of students composing the Medical Class of the University. A copy will, therefore, be placed at your disposal. Accept the assurances of my respect,
> And believe me truly yours, &c.,
> SAMUEL JACKSON.[3]

Portions of three lectures given to Brice's class, as well as the commencement address to the graduates of 1851, illustrate the education of medical students in Philadelphia—from both the North and the South—a decade before the Civil War. Presentations during the autumn term of 1850 include those by **George Bacon Wood** (*Introductory to the course of lectures on the theory and practice of medicine, in the University of Pennsylvania, delivered October 11, 1850,* Philadelphia, Merrihew and Thompson, Printers, published by the class, 1850), **Samuel Jackson** (*An introductory lecture, preliminary to a course on the Institutes of Medicine, delivered on the 9th of October, 1850, before the class of the University of Pennsylvania,* Philadelphia, Journeymen Printers' Office, No. 5 Harmony Court, published by the class, 1850), and **Joseph Carson** (*Lecture Introductory to the course on materia medica and pharmacy in the University of Pennsylvania, delivered October 10, 1850,* Philadelphia, Merrihew and Thompson, Printers, published by the class, 1850). Excerpts by Wood and Jackson appear below; Carson's material appears in Appendix X.

Professor Wood acknowledges that members of the medical profession are not all knowing, and should strive to expand knowledge:

> Do we profess to have secret depths which ordinary intellect cannot fathom? Do we claim certainty or universality of knowledge, or infallibility of judgment? Or rather, do we not profess openly that our science is yet imperfect?—that, though much has been learned, yet much still remains to be learned?—that though we can do much good, we cannot do all good? Do we not proclaim that we seek only for truth; that we are open to its reception

Appendix XII

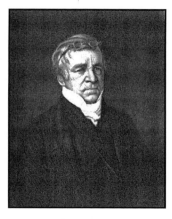

Figure 1, left
Nathaniel Chapman, M.D. (1780–1853)

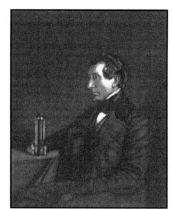

Figure 2, right
William E. Horner, M.D. (1793–1853)

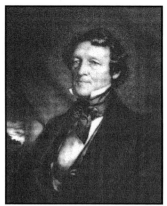

Figure 3, left
George B. Wood, M.D. (1797–1879)

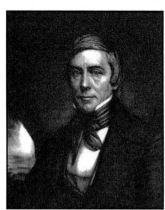

Figure 4, right
James B. Rogers, M.D. (1802–1852)

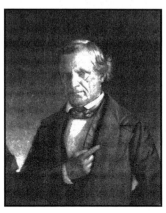

Figure 5, left
William Gibson, M.D. (1788–1868)

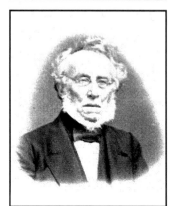

Figure 6, right
Hugh L. Hodge, M.D. (1796–1873)

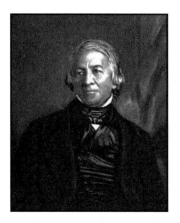

Figure 7, left
Samuel Jackson, M.D. (1787–1872)

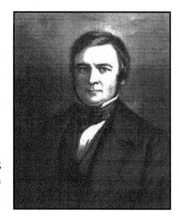

Figure 8, right
Joseph Carson, M.D. (1808–1876)

from whatever source it may come; and that our greatest zeal is to enlarge the boundaries of our knowledge, and the extent of our capacity of usefulness?[4]

He apprises the students of quacks, and attributes their "successes" to the tendency of some diseases to be self-limited:

> It is true that most diseases, if left to themselves, and sometimes even under positively injurious treatment, will sooner or later terminate favorably, through the inherent powers of the…[patient]. Hence the frequent apparent success of irregular and unskillful practitioners. It is in fact on this basis, and on the prevalent ignorance of the truth just stated, that the whole edifice of quackery, in all its forms, mainly rests. … The…[charlatan] knows that a disease will in all probability end favorably within a certain time, and, administering his nostrum, claims the result as a proof of his own skill.[5]

Dr. Wood could have told them also that their own "successful" outcomes might not reflect their treatment, but instead the natural history of a patient's illness, but he does not. His students are taught at the outset that the study of medicine is a lifelong process: "You will learn, before many years, that your graduation in medicine is simply the era at which you are to begin your own self-guidance in the pursuit of professional knowledge.…[6]

Dr. Wood lauds the "enormous body" of medical knowledge collected by 1850, but urges his students to question its accuracy and how it is acquired:

> May it not be that all this vast amount of knowledge is mere useless lore… Of the immense value of medical knowledge, if it is what it purports to be, there can be but one opinion. To relieve pain, to save life, to preserve health; these are aims, which can scarcely be overstated. The question, then, is, does a knowledge of medicine, as at present taught, really contribute toward those great results, which are its professed aim and end?
>
> To answer this question rationally we must have recourse to the two great principles by which truth is tested; to…**judgment**…and to **experience**. [emphasis added]. From the beginning of history…men, among the first certainly in mental powers and attainments, have devoted themselves to the observation of disease, and to the recording of the facts observed. While the process of collection has thus been going on, the accumulated material has been…subjected to a careful scrutiny, and the false and useless…separated, thrown aside, and forgotten. The medical knowledge of the present times is thus the slow growth of centuries, …during which, as in the growth of living bodies, an intellectual digestion and nutrition have been going on, the useless and effete being thrown off at the same time that the useful and efficient has been assimilated…, the latter…constantly increasing…, until our science shall become mature, and nature have yielded to human investigation all that she possesses of the preservative and remedial.[7]

Wood tells them that science is based on making a hypothesis about a problem, questioning the evidence, and judging which is the correct answer:

Appendix XII

> Imaginative minds in our profession have from time to time put forth hypotheses—many of them...futile, many with but partial glimpses into yet undiscovered truths; but these are received for what they are worth, examined, sifted, and partially or wholly rejected, as they prove to be more or less founded in truth, or altogether baseless."[8]

Wood's pronouncements sound modern, but **judgment** is not how medical science, or any other science, derives truth; instead it is by experimentation in the laboratory. His other method for discovering how disease occurs or whether treatment is effective is **experience**:

> To the practitioner...the proofs of the efficacy of his measures are too frequently offered to admit of doubt. Every day he witnesses cases of suffering in which relief follows almost immediately the use of appropriate remedies. Chronic affections frequently came under his notice, which, after a long course of steady deterioration, with no hope of spontaneous amendment, commence a course of amelioration from the moment that the influence of treatment is felt, and it often happens that the period at which benefit will accrue may be confidently predicted. It is his great happiness to believe that, in not a few instances, fatal results are averted through his instrumentality.[8]

Professor Wood cites examples of "successful" treatments with iron, foxglove, baking powder, mercury, and arsenic, which the students will observe in patients admitted to the Pennsylvania Hospital (established 1751) and to the Philadelphia Hospital (descended from the Philadelphia Almshouse, built 1731–1732; called the Philadelphia Hospital in 1835; eventually named the Philadelphia General Hospital;[9] closed in 1977):

> For yourselves, my young friends, ...[in] the wards of our hospitals...you...have the opportunity of seeing patients, who had been gradually becoming worse and worse for weeks or months, or who...had been suffering for years, beginning to improve under the means employed, and regularly going on to health, often at the very time, and in the very manner predicted by the prescriber. The bloodless young woman, with her palpitating heart, her embarrassed breathing, and nervous symptoms of extreme violence, is put on the use of the preparations of iron, and, in from 3 to 6 weeks, leaves the hospital, rosy, cheerful, and in full health. The bloated, dropsically [swollen, edematous] patient, whose disease had been slowly advancing for months, takes his foxglove [digitalis], or cream of tartar...and rapidly recovers under its influence. Every variety of chronic inflammation you behold yielding to the careful administration of mercury. Skin diseases, which have been the misery of their victim for years...vanish before your eyes under the use of arsenical preparations.[10]

Typical of medical practice of the time, experience is the major arbiter of successful treatment. As pointed out in Chapter II, James Lind's controlled trial of 1753 using citrus fruit and other substances to treat scurvy is not mentioned in these lectures. Similarly, Pierre C. A. Louis' studies on the influence of bleeding or not bleeding patients with pneumonia and other diseases in 1836 are absent from lectures heard by Brice and his fellow students. "Bad air" as a cause of several diseases figures prominently, however, and requires ventilation and avoidance of "morbific [disease-causing] effluvia [malodorous vapors, gases], whether from crowded human beings or from paludal [malarial] sources."[11]

Dr. G. B. Wood emphasizes that the goal of the University of Pennsylvania School of Medicine is to do whatever it takes to teach their students well, in this case extending its course of study from four to six months:

> This was, in fact, nothing more than was necessary to keep us from retrograding from that position which, as a school, it has been our ambition to maintain. The science of medicine has been greatly enlarged within the last fifty years; and to teach it as thoroughly as it was taught before that period requires a longer time.[12]

Professor Wood directs the students to prepare "for the fearful encounter with disease to follow." Lectures will teach them "the most characteristic and most important points of each subject," but students are directed to learn "minute details...[from] published treatises and private study."[13] Essentially this meant going to the library of the College of Physicians of Philadelphia, the nation's oldest honorary medical academy (1787), since the University of Pennsylvania did not have a medical library until 1931.[14]

Wood plans to supplement their teaching with his observations and with illustrations and models:

> Along with the prominent and peculiar features of the several diseases, in all their different relations, I propose to give you the results of my own personal observation, reflection, and experience, so as to render the course in some degree characteristic. Another object will be to make the lectures as demonstrative as possible by introducing illustrative representations, such as morbid preparations, drawings, models, etc.; in this way appealing to the eye as well as the ear, and seeking an entrance into the understanding and memory by two avenues instead of one. To enable me to fulfil [sic] this latter purpose, I made during the summer...a voyage to Europe; and I am happy to inform the class that it has not been altogether fruitless. I have already received a considerable amount of illustrative material....[15]

He ends by expressing his feelings about their medical school and about medicine of the time.

> As an institution, I can say proudly, apart from any personal concern, that we deserve success. It has been, and continues to be our great aim to maintain medical education, at the highest point of which it is susceptible among us, and thus to contribute at once to the elevation of the character of our beloved profession, and to one of the highest temporal interests of our no less beloved country.[16]

Walter Brice and his classmates have been in medical school only three days of their fall term, and already are being made aware of the prestige associated with the University of Pennsylvania School of Medicine, the country's oldest medical school, founded in 1765. Professor Samuel Jackson (1787–1872), M.D. from the University of Pennsylvania School of Medicine, 1812, greets them:

Appendix XII

> GENTLEMEN MEDICAL STUDENTS:
>
> I salute you and welcome you to this ancient seat of medical science and instruction.
>
> The University from its foundation has been devoted to the maintaining of the honor and dignity of the profession, to the cultivation of medicine as a science, to the expansion and perfecting of its instruction, keeping pace with advancing knowledge.
>
> The Faculty feel the responsibility that rests on them, and will omit no endeavor to hold up the well-earned renown of the school. The instruction of the courses will be kept on a level with the progress of the times; sound principles and correct practice will be enforced, and a high professional tone be infused in the students....[17]

Jackson gives the future doctors a perspective of the profession:

> The object you propose to yourselves in coming to this city is laudable; the motives that govern your selection of medicine as a profession are noble. You would be physicians—men-healers—men-savers. It is in the order of Providence that all that live must suffer and die. None are exempt from this universal law. ...While suffering, disease, and death are knitted with the life-yarn of man into his existence, yet is there much of each wholly avoidable, ...which may be prevented, and from which he may be saved.[18]

He defines the scope of medicine in society and in the sciences, and what the class must study to enter it:

> This knowledge, which covers an immense field and involves a great amount of research, constitutes the science and practice of medicine. It must form, in the organization of society, the pursuit of an exclusive profession, devoted to the investigation of man's...life, in all their various modes, states, conditions, and phases of existence. The range of studies embraced in the medical profession is the whole of the physiological sciences, those especially that have relation immediately to the physical, vital, and moral nature of man, in health and in disease.[19]

Jackson expounds on medicine as a science, but not one of the "exact" sciences like astronomy or chemistry:

> I propose, as the subject of this discourse, to show to you that medicine is a science and not a mere art; a combination of scientific and philosophical laws, and... requires for its exercise extensive knowledge, intelligence, and judgment.
>
> There are, philosophically speaking, no accidents, no chance in nature.
>
> **Throughout her vast domains the supremacy of law prevails; harmony and order reign** [emphasis his]. No operation, no phenomenon occurs...that is not the result of a pre-existing law. The sciences to which the term exact is

Excerpts from Lectures

> applied, afford the most apt...illustration. In astronomy phenomena are determined with the utmost precision, to the smallest fractions of time. This may be done not only for the present, but may be carried far into the past, or be extended into the infinity of the future. The certainty of astronomical science arises from the simpleness [sic] of its facts, and the unity of its laws—the one consisting of the movements of the great masses of matter forming the heavenly bodies, and the other, the Newtonian law, the cause of those movements.[20]

He extols the exactness of chemistry and the advances made possible by the other physical sciences:

> Chemical science, though far more complicated in its phenomena and laws, falls very little short of astronomy in the accuracy of its processes and its calculations. The chemist performs his experiment with almost unerring certainty. He knows positively what results will occur by bringing together different chemical substances. He can give the exact components of a mineral substance from its crystalline form, found in any part of the world. [Chemists] follow rules and formulae.... Chemistry, by its researches, has penetrated to the molecules of matter. It weighs them, ascertains their numbers in any body, studies their properties, affinities, and other relations. These are so accurately ascertained, that they are arranged into tables for reference; Chemistry, in modern times, rivals Mathematics and Geometry in the exactness of its calculations and the precision of its formulae.[21]

Jackson describes medical science, by contrast, as an inexact science:

> The physiological or medical...sciences have no such character. The phenomena are complicated, not one is simple and single. Viewed superficially, the phenomena of the Physiological and Medical sciences appear unstable, confused, complex, and obscure, exposed to a thousand chances and subject to endless accidents.[22]

He also tells them that a life force is needed to direct the functions of the body. Actions in living things are "directed by a special law; it is an organic or life law. Now these life...actions, and this life...law, are not manifested except under the acting of a force, —it is...[a] life-force."[23] The idea of the life force (called vitalism) was that only living things could create organic compounds. As noted in Chapter II, vitalism persisted until the end of the American Civil War, when Claude Bernard demonstrated that physical and chemical reactions alone permitted all the body's functions to occur, and did not require any mysterious invisible vital force to do so.

Like Professor George Wood, Dr. Jackson attributes disease to "bad," "mal," or "poisonous" air. Concerning sources of "contamination of the air," Jackson says it occurs by:

> Exhalations from manufactories, by various processes of the arts, and by fermentation and putrefaction. The soil of the earth is a vast compost of decaying animal and vegetable matters, the products of which...are exhaled into the air, infecting it with malarial and other poisons, scattering broadcast the seeds of disease and death.[24]

Appendix XII

Jackson next states that medicines have specific actions on various organs and can be classified by these actions:

> In therapeutics, ...[there is] a special relation between...medicinal substances and particular organs...through which the vital state of the organs and the operations of their functions are modified.
>
> These relations are so regular, that medicines are arranged, in the materia medica, in particular classes, designated by names expressive of the influences they exert on the whole...[patient], or on certain organs and functions, as sedatives, stimulants, emetics, purgatives, &c. The articles of these classes are prescribed with a strong assurance that, if judiciously selected and administered, the effects expressed in the name will be realized.[25]

Appendix X lists the most common classification of medications in use in the latter half of the nineteenth century.

Dr. Jackson closes his lecture with these optimistic and inspiring words:

> In the manner in which the subjects discussed in this discourse have been handled, you will have seen the mode which is pursued in my course. Physiological phenomena are analyzed—are reduced to their simplest elements; they are studied in their origin, as to their offices in the economy and relations with each other. I feel sensibly that my powers are inadequate to the performance, in the way I could wish, of this important task. But should I succeed in inspiring you with a love of science, and of exciting in you a determination to accomplish yourselves as scientific physicians, the interpreters of God's organic laws for the preservation of health, the assuaging of suffering, and alleviation of man's physical evils, I shall have performed the obligations imposed on me, conferred, through you, a benefit on society, and gratified the height of my ambition.[26]

Finally, the commencement address delivered to Walter Brice and his classmates on April 5, 1851, by their Professor of Anatomy and Dean of the medical school, William E. Horner, allows us another glimpse into the training of pre-Civil War physicians, as well as society's expectations of them after graduation. Horner addresses four distinct parties present at the ceremony:

> 1. To the audience I am introducing...young gentlemen who have distinguished themselves in their studies, and obtained corresponding honors. 2. To the Graduates of the occasion I have to give those precepts, on which the good and the wise are all of common consent. 3. To the constituted authorities and guardians of this ancient Institution, I am to report how far the trust committed to its Medical Faculty has been executed in the spirit of its appointment. 4. And to the collective assemblage, I have to exhibit the tendencies and policy of a School of Medicine which has occupied uninterruptedly, a large share of public confidence and attention...for nearly a century—a period certainly distant in its inception, when compared with what we see around us, of men and of things, in this most progressive and favored of countries.[27]

He attests to the graduates' "unremitted [sic] ardor and attention in the prosecution of their studies..." and their "irreproachable and urbane conduct...," and says that the University of Pennsylvania "confidently looks forward to the period when these, the youngest of her children, will be amongst the brightest of her ornaments, and serve also to perpetuate her reputation." He states that "careful examination and inquiry by the Medical Faculty into their qualifications...has satisfied the Faculty that...their proficiency in medicine is such, that the interests and dignity of the science are safe with them—and that the lives of the people may be confided to their care."[28]

Dr. Horner addresses the graduates:

> Your recent studies, gentlemen, have presented to you...an exposition of the structure and functions of the human frame—of the diseases and perversions of action to which it is liable, and of the resources furnished by botany, chemistry, pharmacy, and the principles of medical practice, to arrest its disorders, and to re-instate it in its healthy action. It may not be apparent to you now, but the time will come when you will join in the general sentiment of the advanced members of the profession, that the best conducted medical education leaves much to be acquired at the subsequent periods of life.[29]

Concerning their teachers, Horner comments, "In the courses of instruction which you have just terminated, many of the ideas which have been imparted to you in one hour of lecturing, are the results of weeks of toil and of reflection on the part of your teachers."[30]

He addresses their responsibilities regarding continuous postgraduate education and adding to the body of medical knowledge:

> There is unquestionably no profession which requires a more intimate acquaintance with its rules of practice and with its materials, than medicine. Cases of sudden emergency are constantly arising in which the self-possession of the practitioner is the only barrier between the patient and death—the slightest confusion of mind or agitation of hand becomes the turning point of safety. Every one should prepare himself for scenes of this kind, for there are none of us who have been engaged to any extent in the practice of medicine, who have not been called upon to take a part in them. Besides a revision and a supplementary course of study, it is also incumbent on you to be a diligent observer of what is passing around, and to increase your stock of knowledge by a liberal intercourse with the most intelligent members of your profession, and by a perusal of the most esteemed medical periodicals and works of the day.[31]

Horner speaks to medical ethics:

> Not unfrequently [sic] the most secret concerns of families are exposed to him either by accident or through deliberative action. No physician can safely make a habit of speaking, even on the indifferent concerns of the families he visits.... It is scarcely necessary for me to say that information acquired through professional channels and confidence, should have a seal as solemn as that of death put upon it; and that neither fine nor imprisonment, nor torture should have influence enough to make the physician break this seal.[32]

Appendix XII

He reflects that when the life of a physician whose life was "thus well spent…" came to an end, he would feel "as if his mission had been properly accomplished, and that usefulness to others being its great and redeeming object, he had lived not for himself alone but for the comfort and happiness of those around him."[33] Horner comments further, "With the time appropriated to his practice, to his studies, and to his notes, no physician can devote much to the ordinary pleasures and pursuits of life."[34]

To the "gentlemen Trustees, the dignified and the estimable guardians of this ancient corporation…," he extols Dr. George Bacon Wood as giving the medical school's department of Theory and Practice of Medicine "a position unrivalled in any part of the world." Specifically he refers to Dr. Wood's publication, *Treatise on the Practice of Medicine*, editions in 1847 and 1849, as "unequalled in popularity by any which went before it either here or in Europe."[35] Professor Horner reviews the academic year just ending:

> The session for 1850–51 opened on Monday, October 7th. The first week having been given up to introductory, the lectures began regularly on the 14th of the same month, and with the exception of a holiday for a week at Christmas, were continued uninterruptedly till the last week of March, 1851. Our lectures, in occupying twenty-two weeks…presented a curriculum, including hospital instruction, of about **seven hundred and four lectures of one hour each** [emphasis added], a duration we believe much in advance of the curriculum of any other in the country.[36]

Lastly, Horner contrasts medical education in Europe with that in the U.S.: "The course of education on the continent of Europe is widely different from our own; from five to seven years of study…are demanded, [whereas in the United States]…a Doctor of Medicine… [is] made in eighteen months…."[37] Professor Horner closes thus: "With the above views, my young friends, I now take an affectionate adieu. May you henceforth enjoy all the advantages of time so well devoted to your studies."[38]

Credentials of those who taught Walter Brice follow: **James B. Rogers** (1802–1852) wrote *Elements of chemistry* in 1846, an 848-page textbook. **William Gibson** (1788–1868) wrote eight editions of *Institutes and Practice of Surgery* between 1824–1845. He comprised List of Physicians in the U.S. in 1836. Gibson traveled to Europe, recording his experiences there in an 1841 publication, *Rambles in Europe in 1839*. Professor Gibson achieved distinction also by delivering two babies with the same mother by Caesarean section. Schroeder-Lein says that only seventy-nine such procedures were performed in the United States between 1822 and 1877.[39] **Hugh L. Hodge** (1796–1873) was a prolific author. His *Principles and practice of obstetrics*, a work of 550 pages, was published in 1864. Two years later appeared *The principles and practice of obstetrics: illustrated with one hundred and fifty-nine lithographic figures from original photographs, and with numerous woodcuts*. In addition he wrote two editions of a 500-page work, *On diseases peculiar to women: including displacements of the uterus*, in 1860 and 1868. **Nathaniel Chapman** (1780–1853) published on a variety of medical topics: *On midwifery and diseases of women and children* (1810), *Dropsy and angina pectoris, with dissections* (1820), *Gout and rheumatism* (1844), and several editions of *History and improvement of the materia medica* (1821–1831). **Joseph Carson** (1808–1876) was Professor of *Materia Medica* at the University of Pennsylvania School of Medicine during the 1850s and 1860s, and had as his predecessor, since 1835, **George Bacon Wood**. Wood (1797–1879), with Franklin Bache, published at least ten editions of the *Dispensatory of the United States of*

America between 1833 and 1858. George Bacon Wood (1797–1879), well traveled, went on a medical tour of Europe and of St. Petersburg [Russia], which he reported to his students during a lecture on October 14, 1853. **Samuel Jackson** (1787–1872) received his M.D. degree from the University of Pennsylvania School of Medicine in 1812. He published at least 36 works between 1808 and 1859, on such topics as cholera, yellow fever, and principles of medicine. He was also active in the Philadelphia Medical Society. **William E. Horner** (1793–1853) traveled to Germany to examine medical training, facilities, and treatment, which he shared in great detail with his students in 1848. During the same trip he visited Paris, where he witnessed an insurrection that resulted in many battle wounds. From Horner's Paris experience, his students hear the following, perhaps the only account presaging the wounds of war that they will encounter just over a decade later:

> The Hotel Dieu is the most eminent of the French Hospitals for Clinical Surgery [italics in original]. I was therefore anxious to see the state and treatment of the wounded there; it was also immediately in the vicinity of some of the most sanguinary of the insurgent operations. Its wards were filled with the wounded, generally injured by musket balls, and having a very large proportion of extremely severe inflictions. Bones shattered to pieces; joints perforated; the great cavities opened; the face sadly torn; a few limbs amputated, which had occurred during or immediately after the action. The treatment I found to be very much the same as with us, in regard to local applications. It consisted, for the most part, of flaxseed poultices applied warm in the severer cases; those of less severity received as a dressing…of lint spread with cerate [wax]. Some few cases had the cold water treatment, or that by irrigation, in allowing a small stream of water to keep well moistened some layers of linen laid over the wounds.[40]

Resources available to the class of Walter Brice were numerous. In addition to anatomic models (similar ones can be seen at the Mütter Museum in Philadelphia, contributed by surgeon Thomas Dent Mütter from Jefferson Medical College), the class had access to several microscopes, and some medical journals at the College of Physicians of Philadelphia, which served as the medical library for the University of Pennsylvania's students until 1931.[41]

The class would probably have read the *Journal of the American Medical Association, JAMA*. The association was founded in 1847. By January of 1848 the first volume, called then the Transactions of the AMA, was in print. The medical students would not have a medical index, however, facilitating location of current medical literature. The first one revolutionized the ability of physicians to exchange and share medical information. Not surprisingly, the large surgical and anesthesia experience of the Civil War provided the impetus to create such an index. Begun in 1880, it was printed by the Government Printing Office in Washington, D.C., and called the *Catalogue of the Library of the Surgeon General's Office U.S. Army*. It arranged publications by author and by subject, and was published until 1961.

Titles of theses written by the class of 1851, required for the doctor of medicine degree, may be found in Appendix II, grouped by topic. All titles except that of William H. Denny, of Ellicott's Mills, MD, are listed in the Commencement Program of April 5, 1851. There were 167 students in the class.

Appendix XII

Appendix XII References

1. *Catalogue of the Trustees, Officers & Students of the University of Pennsylvania, Session 1849–50.* Philadelphia: L.R. Bailey, Printer; 1850: 8
2. *Catalogue of the Trustees, Officers & Students of the University of Pennsylvania, Session 1850–51.* Philadelphia: L.R. Bailey, Printer; 1851: 8
3. Jackson S. *An introductory lecture, preliminary to a course on the Institutes of Medicine, delivered on the 9th of October, 1850, before the class of the University of Pennsylvania.* Philadelphia: Journeymen Printers' Office; 1850.
4. Wood GB. *Introductory to the course of lectures on the theory and practice of medicine, in the University of Pennsylvania, delivered October 11, 1850.* Philadelphia: Merrihew and Thompson, Printers; 1850:10
5. *Ibid.*, 11–12
6. *Ibid.*, 15
7. *Ibid.*, 8–9
8. *Ibid.*, 10
9. Henry FP, ed. *Founders' Week Memorial Volume published by the City of Philadelphia in Commemoration of the two hundred and twenty-fifth Anniversary of its Founding.* Philadelphia; 1909: 465–516
10. Wood GB. *Introductory to the course of lectures on the theory and practice of medicine, in the University of Pennsylvania, delivered October 11, 1850.* Philadelphia: Merrihew and Thompson, Printers; 1850: 12–13
11. *Ibid.*, 13–14
12. *Ibid.*, 15
13. *Ibid.*, 18
14. Seymour A. Personal communication: 10-8-99
15. Wood GB. *Introductory to the course of lectures on the theory and practice of medicine, in the University of Pennsylvania, delivered October 11, 1850.* Philadelphia: Merrihew and Thompson, Printers; 1850: 19
16. *Ibid.*, 23
17. Jackson S. *An introductory lecture, preliminary to a course on the Institutes of Medicine, delivered on the 9th of October, 1850, before the class of the University of Pennsylvania.* Philadelphia: Journeymen Printers' Office; 1850: 5
18. *Ibid.*, 5–6
19. *Ibid.*, 6
20. *Ibid.*, 6–7
21. *Ibid.*, 6–8
22. *Ibid.*, 8
23. *Ibid.*, 14
24. Jackson S. *An introductory lecture, preliminary to a course on the Institutes of Medicine, delivered on the 9th of October, 1850, before the class of the University of Pennsylvania.* Philadelphia: Journeymen Printers' Office; 1850: 16
25. *Ibid.*, 12–13
26. *Ibid.*, 20
27. Horner WE. *Medical Commencement of the University of Pennsylvania held on Saturday, April 5, 1851: with a Valedictory by W. E. Horner, M.D., Professor of Anatomy.* Philadelphia: L.R. Bailey, Printer; 1851: 11–12
28. *Ibid.*, 12
29. *Ibid.*, 12–13

30. *Ibid.*, 13
31. *Ibid.*, 14
32. *Ibid.*, 17–18
33. *Ibid.*, 18
34. *Ibid.*, 15
35. *Ibid.*, 22
36. *Ibid.*, 25
37. *Ibid.*, 29
38. *Ibid.*, 32
39. Schroeder-Lein, G. *Confederate Hospitals on the Move*. Columbia, SC: University of South Carolina Press; 1994: 32
40. Horner WE. *Introductory Lecture before the Anatomical Class of the University of Pennsylvania, delivered October 17, 1848*. Philadelphia: T.K. and P.G. Collins, printers; 1848: 11–12
41. Bell WJ, Jr. *The College of Physicians of Philadelphia, a Bicentennial History*. Canton, MA: Science History Publications; 1987: 11

Bibliography

Books

Alley G. *Observations on the Hydrargyria; or that vesicular disease arising from the exhibition of mercury.* London: Whittingham and Rowland, for Longman, Hurst, Rees, and Orme; 1810

Bannatyne GA. *Rheumatoid arthritis: its pathology, morbid anatomy, and treatment.* Bristol: John Wright; 1896

Bayne-Jones S. *The evolution of preventive medicine in the U.S. Army, 1607–1939.* Washington: US Government Printing Office; 1968

Beck J. *Essays on Infant therapeutics: to which are added Observations on Ergot, and an Account of the Origin of the use of Mercury in Inflammatory Complaints.* New York: W. E. Dean; 1849

Bell WJ, Jr. *The College of Physicians of Philadelphia, a Bicentennial History.* Canton, MA: Science History Publications; 1987

Bengtson BP, Kuz, JE. *Photographic Atlas of Civil War Injuries.* Grand Rapids, Michigan: Medical Staff Press, in association with Kennesaw, GA: Kennesaw Mountain Press, Inc.; 1996

Bernard C, Hutted C. *Illustrated manual of operative surgery and surgical anatomy.* New York: Billiard Brothers; 1861

Bollet AJ. *Civil War Medicine Challenges and Triumphs.* Tucson, AZ: Galen Press, Ltd.; 2002

Carson J. *Synopsis of the Course of Lectures on Materia Medica and Pharmacy, Delivered in the University of Pennsylvania.* Philadelphia: Blanchard and Lea; 1851

Cavanaugh J. *Historical Sketch of the Obion Avalanche, Company H, Ninth Tennessee Infantry, Confederate States of America.* Union City, TN: The Commercial; 1922

Cecil Textbook of Medicine, Wyngaarden JB, Smith LH, Jr., eds., 18th ed. Philadelphia: W.B. Saunders Co.; 1988

Chisholm JJ. *A manual of military surgery, for the use of surgeons in the Confederate Army.* Charleston SC: Evans & Cogswell; 1861

Dammann G. *Pictorial Encyclopedia of Civil War Medical Instruments and Equipment.* Missoula, MT: Pictorial Publishing Co.; Volume I (1983); Volume II (1988); Volume III (1997)

Daniel LJ. *Shiloh: The Battle That Changed the Civil War.* New York: Simon & Schuster; 1997

Denney RE. *Civil War Medicine: Care & Comfort of the Wounded.* New York: Sterling Publishing Co., Inc.; 1995

Desmond K. *A Timetable of Inventions and Discoveries.* New York: M. Evans & Co.; 1986

Dictionary of Scientific Biography, ed. Gillispie CC. Charles Scribner's Sons, NY; 1981

Documents of the U.S. Sanitary Commission. New York: U.S. Sanitary Commission; 1866

Dorwart BB. *Carson's Materia Medica: An Annotation.* Bala Cynwyd, PA: WVD Press; 2003

Dunglison R. *A Dictionary of Medical Science*, 6th ed. Philadelphia: Lea and Blanchard; 1846

Felsen J. *Bacillary Dysentery Colitis and Enteritis.* Philadelphia: W.B. Saunders Co.; 1945

Flannery MA. *Civil War Pharmacy: A History of Drugs, Drug Supply and Provision, and Therapeutics for the Union and Confederacy.* Binghamton, NY: Hayworth Press, Inc.; 2004

Fleming JR. *The Ninth Tennessee Infantry: a Roster.* Shippensburg, PA: White Mane Publishing Co.; 1996

Flexner A. *Medical Education in the United States and Canada.* Boston: D.B. Updike, Merrymount Press; 1910

Forrester RC. *Glory and Tears: Obion County, Tennessee 1860–1870.* Union City, TN: H.A. Lanzer Co.; 1966

Founders' Week Memorial Volume published by the City of Philadelphia in Commemoration of the two hundred and twenty-fifth Anniversary of its Founding, Henry FP, ed. Philadelphia; 1909

Freemon FR. *Microbes and Minie Balls: An Annotated Bibliography of Civil War Medicine.* Cranbury, NJ: Associated University Presses, Inc.; 1993

Garrod, AB. *A Treatise on Gout and Rheumatic Gout (Rheumatoid Arthritis).* London: Longmans, Green; 1876

Goodman L, Gilman A. *The Pharmacological Basis of Therapeutics*, 5th ed. New York: Macmillan Publishing Co., Inc.; 1975

Habershon SO. *On the injurious effects of mercury in the treatment of disease.* London: John Churchill; 1840

Hamilton FH. A practical treatise on military surgery. New York: Billiard Brothers; 1861

Harrison's Principles of Internal Medicine, ed. Fauci AS, 15th ed. New York: McGraw-Hill; 1998

Horner WE. *Introductory Lecture before the Anatomical Class of the University of Pennsylvania, delivered October 17, 1848.* Philadelphia: T.K. and P.G. Collins, printers; 1848

Horner WE. *Medical Commencement of the University of Pennsylvania held on Saturday, April 5, 1851: with a Valedictory by W. E. Horner, M.D., Professor of Anatomy.* Philadelphia: L.R. Bailey, Printer; 1851

Infectious Diseases, ed. Hoeprich PD, 2nd ed. Hagerstown, MD: Harper and Row; 1977

Infectious Diseases, eds. Hoeprich PD, Jordan MC, Ronald AR, 5th ed. Philadelphia: J.B. Lippincott Co.; 1994

Jackson S. *An introductory lecture, preliminary to a course on the Institutes of Medicine, delivered on the 9th of October, 1850, before the class of the University of Pennsylvania.* Philadelphia: Journeymen Printers' Office; 1850

Jones J. *Medical and Surgical Memoirs 1855–1876.* New Orleans: Clark and Hofeline; 1876

Jones J. *Suggestions on Medical Education. Introductory Lecture to the course of 1859–60 in the Medical College of Georgia.* Augusta, GA: Constitutionalist Book and Job Office; 1860

Letterman J. *Medical Recollections of the Army of the Potomac.* New York: Appleton and Co.; 1866

Bibliography

Lind's Treatise on Scurvy. Reprint of the first edition of James Lind of 1753, ed. Stewart CP, Guthrie D. Edinburgh: Edinburgh University Press; 1953

Mandell, Douglas, and Bennett's Principles and Practice of Infectious Diseases, eds. Mandell GL, Bennett JE, Dolin R, 6th ed. Philadelphia: Elsevier Churchill Livingstone, Inc.; 2005

Manual of Surgery, eds. Cooper A, Green JH. New York: Thomas Castle (Charles S. Francis); 1839

Medical and Surgical History of the Civil War. Wilmington, NC: Broadfoot Publishing; 1990

Medical and Surgical History of the War of the Rebellion (1861–65). Washington, DC: Government Printing Office; 1888

Merck's Manual of the Materia Medica, 1st ed. New York: Merck and Co.; 1899

Military Medical and Surgical Essays prepared for the USSC, ed. Hammond, WA. Philadelphia: J.B. Lippincott and Co.; 1864

Moore SP. Regulations of the Confederate States of America Medical Department, in *Regulations for the Army of the Confederate States.* Richmond: Randolph; 1862. Repub.: San Francisco: Norman Publishing; 1992

Morton LT, Moore RJ. *A Chronology of Medicine and Related Sciences.* Brookfield, VT: Ashgate; 1997

Netter. FH. *Ciba Collection of Medical Illustrations, Digestive System,* Vol. 3. West Caldwell, NJ: Ciba; Part I (1959); Part II (1962)

Ordronaux J. *Manual of Instructions for Military Surgeons.* NY: D. Van Nostrand; 1863

Principles and Practice of Infectious Diseases, eds. Mandell GL, Douglas RG, Jr., Bennett, JE, 3rd ed. New York: Churchill Livingstone; 1990

Reply of the judge advocate, John A. Bingham, to the defence of the accused, before a general court-martial for the trial of Brig. Gen. William A. Hammond, Surgeon General, USA. Washington: Govt. Printing Office; 1864

Rutkow IM. *The History of Surgery in the United States 1775–1900.* San Francisco: Norman Publishing; Volume I (1988); Volume II (1992)

Rutkow IM. *Bleeding Blue and Gray: Civil War Surgery and the Evolution of American Medicine.* New York: Random House; 2005

Schaadt MJ. *Civil War Medicine—an Illustrated History.* Quincy, Illinois: Cedarwood Publishing; 1998

Schroeder-Lein, G. *Confederate Hospitals on the Move.* Columbia, SC: University of South Carolina Press; 1994

Shattuck L. *Report of a General Plan for the promotion of public and personal health.* Boston: Dutton and Wentworth; 1850

Smith S. *Hand-book of surgical operations.* New York: Billiard Brothers; 1862

Stedman's Medical Dictionary, 26th ed. Baltimore: Williams & Wilkins; 1995

Steiner PE. *Disease in the Civil War.* Springfield, IL: Charles C. Thomas; 1968

Stillé A. *Therapeutics and Materia Medica,* Vol. II. Philadelphia: Blanchard and Lea; 1860

Sutherland DE. *Seasons of War: The Ordeal of a Confederate Community 1861–1865.* Baton Rouge, LA: Louisiana State University Press; 1995

The Whole Works of that excellent Physician, Dr. Thomas Sydenham, Pechey J, ed., 7th ed. London: M. Wellington; 1717

Turner GL'E. *Scientific Instruments 1500–1900.* London: Philip Wilson Publishers; 1998

Webster's New Twentieth Century Dictionary of the English Language Unabridged, 2nd edition. New York: World Publishing Co.; 1964

Wood GB. *Introductory to the course of lectures on the theory and practice of medicine, in the University of Pennsylvania, delivered October 11, 1850.* Philadelphia: Merrihew and Thompson, Printers; 1850

Woodward JJ. *Outlines of the Chief Camp Diseases.* Philadelphia: J.B. Lippincott & Co.; 1863

Wunderlich C. *Das Verhalten der Eigenwärme in Krankheiten [The Temperature in Diseases];* 1868

Journals, Associations and Articles

Acute Rheumatic Fever at a Navy Training Center—San Diego, CA. *Morbidity and Mortality Weekly Report.* 1988

Ahvonen P, Sievers K, Aho, K. Arthritis associated with *Yersinia enterocolitica* Infection. *Acta Rheum Scand.* 1969

Bigelow HJ. Anaesthetic Agents, their mode of exhibition and physiological effects. *Trans AMA* Vol. I. 1848

Brice JM. Tribute to Dr. Walter Brice on the event of his Death. Union City, TN: *The News Banner.* November 9, 1895

Campbell A. Fatal Effects of Calomel. *The India Jour. of Med. Sci.*, Vol. I. 1834

Catalogue of the Trustees, Officers & Students of the University of Pennsylvania, Session 1849–50. Philadelphia: L.R. Bailey, Printer. 1850

Catalogue of the Trustees, Officers & Students of the University of Pennsylvania, Session 1850–51. Philadelphia: L.R. Bailey, Printer. 1851

Cheadle WB. Harveian lectures on the various manifestations of the rheumatic state as exemplified in childhood and early life. *Lancet.* 1889

Cooper A. Gonorrheal Rheumatism, *Lancet.* 1824

Crandon JH et al. Experimental Human Scurvy. *N Engl J Med.* 1940

Davis AC. *Medical Affairs II, University of Pennsylvania Medical Alumni in the Civil War.* Philadelphia: University of Pennsylvania. Spring, 1961

Ellsworth PW. On the Modus operandi of Medicines. *The Boston Medical and Surgical Journal.* 1845

Evanchick CC, Davis DE, Harrington TM. Tuberculosis of Peripheral Joints: An Often Missed Diagnosis. *J Rheumatol.* 1986

Gordon SC, Lauter CB. Mumps arthritis: a review of the literature. *Rev Infect Dis.* 1984

Hasegawa GR, Hambrecht FT. The Confederate Medical Laboratories. *South Med J. 2003*

Bibliography

Heggie AD. Prevention of Streptococcal Pharyngitis and Acute Rheumatic Fever in Navy and Marine Corps Recruits. *Navy Medicine*. 1998

Ho G, Jr. Septic Arthritis Update. *Bulletin on the Rheumatic Diseases*. 2002

James L, McFarland RB. An epidemic of pharyngitis due to a non-hemolytic group A streptococcus at Lowry Air Force Base. *N Engl J Med*. 1971

Jenner E. An inquiry into the causes and effects of the varioloe vaccinoe, a disease discovered in some of the western counties of England—particularly Gloucestershire, and known by the name of the cowpox, London 1798. *The Vaccine Inquirer*, Vol. I. Baltimore: John D. Toy. 1822

Jones TD. Diagnosis of Rheumatic Fever. *JAMA*. 1944

Kazlow PG, Beyer B, Brandeis G. Polyarthritis as the initial symptom of secondary syphilis: case report and review. *Mount Sinai Journal of Medicine*. 1989

Kean BH, Reilly PC. Malaria—the mime. *Am J Med*. 1976

Kling D. Syphilitic arthritis with effusion. *Am J Med Sci*. 1932

McCarty DJ. Phagocytosis of urate crystals in gouty synovial fluid. *Amer. J.Med. Sci.* 1962

Meeting of the Medical Profession Upon Surgeon General Hammond's Order No. 6. *Cincinnati Med. and Surg. News*, Vol. IV. 1863

Mitchell SW. On the effect of opium and its derivative alkaloids. *Am J Med Sci* N. S. 59. 1870

Noer HR. An "experimental" epidemic of Reiter's Syndrome. *JAMA*. 1966

Reginato A, Schumacher HR, Jimenez S, Maurer K. Synovitis in secondary syphilis. *Arthritis Rheum*. 1979

Rose HM et al. Differential agglutination of normal and sensitized sheep erythrocytes by sera of patients with rheumatoid arthritis. *Proc Soc Exp Biol Med*. 1948

Roster Of The Medical Officers Of The Army Of Tennessee. *Southern Historical Society Papers*. Richmond, VA. 1894

Slawson RG. *Medical Training in the United States Prior to the Civil War*. Tenth Annual Conference on Civil War Medicine, Shepherdstown, WV. Aug. 2–4, 2002

Smith, JW and Sanford JP. Viral arthritis. *Ann Intern Med*. 1967 *Smithsonian*. 2004 (June)

Smyth CJ, Freyberg RH, McEwen C. *History of Rheumatology*. Atlanta, GA: Arthritis Foundation. 1985

Special Writing Group of the Committee on Rheumatic Fever...of the American Heart Association. Guidelines for the diagnosis of rheumatic fever, Jones criteria, 1992 update. *JAMA*. 1992

Waugh MA. Bony symptoms in secondary syphilis. *Brit J Vener Dis*. 1976

Wile U, Senear F. A study of the involvement of the bone and joints in early syphilis. *Am J Med Sci*. 1916

Wöhler F. *Annalen der Physik und Chemie*, 2nd series 12. 1828

Index

abscess 15, 26–27, 29, 31, 60–62, 64, 80, 83–86, 113, 116, 127–129, 131, 144
Aigner, Dr. P. 25
ambulance system 15
American College of Rheumatology 39
American Journal of the Medical Sciences 110
American Rheumatism Association 39
Andersonville 24, 70
anesthesia
    chloroform 19, 110–111, 134–135, 141
    ether 19, 110–111, 119–120, 134, 141
ankylosing spondylitis 37, 40, 54–55, 68, 75
Army Medical Museum 88, 115
arsphenamine 108
autopsy/post-mortem 44–46, 49, 57–58, 60, 84–88

B27 gene 50, 54
bad air 19, 115, 153
Barnes, Surg. Gen. Joseph K. 110
Bernard, Dr. Claude 19, 155
bilious remittent fever 119
Billings, Dr. John Shaw 115
blindness 37, 50, 54
blood-letting (venesection) 18, 139
blue mass/blue pill 87, 89–91, 94
Bollet, Dr. Alfred Jay 115
Boston Medical and Surgical Journal 110
Brice, Dr. Gratien Bertrand (See dedication)
Brice, Dr. Walter (See dedication), *xiii*, 17–19, 86, 112–113, 115, 117, 119, 148–149, 153, 156, 158–159
bronchitis 22, 26–28, 31, 80–82, 88
Brown, Dr. H. E. 25
Bumstead, Dr. Freeman 63–65, 93, 95, 106–107, 130

calomel 89, 94, 96–103, 108, 133, 142
Carson, Dr. Joseph *xiii*, 51, 93, 99, 148–150, 158
Carson's Materia Medica of 1851 140–145
catarrh 26, 31, 80–81
Chapman, Dr. Nathaniel 148, 150, 158
childbed fever 120–121
chlorate of potash 45
chloroform 19, 110–111, 134–135, 141
cholera 119, 159
chorea 40, 41, 43
cinchona 51, 91, 120, 141
colchicine/colchicum 44, 51, 67, 143
College of Physicians of Philadelphia 15
common cold 26, 31, 80–82
Confederate States Medical and Surgical Journal 109
Confederate Surgeon General 109, 115
conjunctivitis 37, 50–52, 132–133
controlled trials 18, 93, 152
cowpox 112–113, 136–138
cynanche 48

dengue 119
diarrhea/dysentery 23, 26–29, 31, 35–40, 44, 50–52, 54, 60, 74, 83–84, 87–89, 93, 99–101, 119, 131
diseases, cardiac 40–46, 48–49, 55, 57, 61, 63, 68, 74, 87, 99, 120, 122, 124–126, 142–143, 152
diseases, childhood 22–23, 25, 28, 45
diseases, rheumatic 39–40, 49–52, 58, 71, 73

Ehrlich, Paul 108
enteric fever 119
erysipelas 60, 84–85, 120
ether 19, 110–111, 119–120, 134, 141

Index

Felsen, Dr. J. 35–37, 136
fevers *xii*, 23, 25–29, 31–32, 35, 38–49, 51, 57–58, 60–61, 65–68, 71, 75, 80, 83–84, 87–93, 99, 113–114, 119–121, 126, 128, 131, 137, 139, 142
flies 23–24, 28, 35–37, 116, 143
food poisoning 23, 35, 50

George Washington University, Department of Medicine 18
germ theory of disease 19, 45, 58, 61, 113, 115, 127
Gibson, Dr. William 148, 150, 158
gonococcal/gonorrheal 38, 40, 50, 58, 62–64, 103, 116, 121, 130–132
gout 26, 38–40, 51, 71–73
Gram, Hans Christian Joachim 61
guaiacum 70

Hammond, Surg. Gen. William Alexander 20, 57, 93, 100–103, 109, 115, 130
hand washing 19, 25, 36–37, 81, 116
HLA–B27 50, 54
Hodge, Dr. Hugh L. 148, 150, 158
Holmes, Dr. Oliver Wendell Sr. 19
Horner, Dr. William E. 148, 150, 156–159

immune reaction 37, 40, 43, 50, 52, 66–67, 75
Index Medicus 111, 115
infection 15, 19, 22–23, 28, 30, 36, 38, 41–42, 45, 47, 49–50, 52, 57, 60–66, 82–86, 106–108, 119–120, 127, 130–132, 136
intermittent fever 70, 90, 119
iritis 50, 52, 54

Jackson, Dr. Samuel 148–150, 154–156, 159
Jefferson Medical College *xiii, xiv*, 110–111, 134–135, 159
Jenner, Dr. Edward 136–137
Jones, Dr. Joseph 19, 24, 29–31
Jones Criteria for Diagnosis of Rheumatic Fever 41

Keen, Dr. William Williams, Jr. 110
Koch, Dr. Robert 19, 45, 58, 61, 113, 127

laboratory 18, 45, 62, 102, 113, 127–128, 152
Lancet 50, 110
laryngoscope 44
Letterman, Dr. Jonathan *xiii*, 15, 23–24, 115
life force 19, 155
Lind, Dr. James 18, 50, 57, 114, 152
Lister, Dr. Joseph 19
London Medical Gazette 110
Louis, Dr. Pierre Charles Alexandre 18, 114, 152

malaria 25, 31–32, 38, 40, 51, 67–69, 71, 87, 90–91, 93, 100, 119–120, 153, 155
Manual of Military Surgery 109
McParlin, Dr. Thomas A. 24
measles 22, 24, 38, 70
Medical and Surgical History of the War of the Rebellion (1861–1865) xiii, 15, 31, 39, 43, 45, 49, 55, 60, 71, 80, 86–88, 90–91, 101, 112, 115–116, 130, 146–147
Medical College of Georgia 18–19
Medical College of South Carolina 18
Medical College of Virginia 18
Medical Department of the Army
  U.S.A. 20, 29, 102–103, 115
  C.S.A. 20–21, 29, 102, 115
  World War II 47
Medical Department of the Tulane University of Louisiana 18
Medical Director of the Army of the Potomac 23
medical education *xiii, xiv*, 18–21, 93, 109–111
Medical officers 20–21, 23, 109–110, 117
Medical School of the College of Philadelphia 18
mercurial gangrene 102
mercurial ointment 95
mercurial pills 94
mercurial purging 100

mercurial toxicity 99
mercurials 64, 87, 95–96, 98, 103, 130, 132
mercuric chloride 94, 99, 103, 120, 132–133
mercuris dulcis 108
mercurous chloride 89, 92, 94, 96, 98, 102–103, 108, 133
mercury *xii*, 16, 31, 66, 87, 89–108, 115, 120, 130, 133, 142–144, 152
    preparations of:
        ammoniated 95, 103, 133
        bichloride of 94, 133
        biniodide of 95
        deutiodide 133
        iodide of 95, 103, 133
        oxide of 103, 107, 133
        oxycyanide 103
        perchloride 133
        red iodide of 95
        salicylate 103
        sulphate 103
        tannate 103
miasmatic fevers 119
Mitchell, Dr. Silas Weir *xiii*, 110, 115
Moore, Surg. Gen. Samuel Preston 20, 29, 109, 115
Morbus Mercuriali 99
Morehouse, Dr. George Read *xiii*, 110
mosquitoes 24–25, 28, 70, 90, 116
mumps 22, 40, 72

National Library of Medicine 115
necropsy 44–46, 49, 57–58, 60, 84–88
New England Journal of Medicine 110
Newberry, Dr. J. S. 25

Ordronaux, Dr. John 44, 57, 62, 71
osteoarthritis 38
Otis, Dr. George A., Jr. *xiii*, 86

Pasteur, Louis 19, 127
penicillin 40, 47–48, 61–63, 82, 84, 116, 127, 132
pernicious fever 119

pneumonia 18, 22, 30–32, 49, 60–62, 86–87, 91, 93, 97–98, 114, 116, 120, 129, 152
Porcher, Francis Peyre 109
Pott's disease 57–58
puerperal fever 120–121

quinine/quinia 31, 45, 51, 67, 70, 84, 87, 89–92, 120, 132

rashes 37, 40, 43, 50, 52–53, 63–66, 88–89, 96, 99–100, 106–107, 113, 119–120
reactive arthritis *xii*, 40, 50, 52–54, 63, 75
remittent fever 119
Resources of the Southern Fields and Forests: Medical, Economical, and Agricultural 109
rheumatic fever *xii*, 31, 38, 40–49, 57, 68, 75, 126, 128
rheumatic ophthalmia 50–51
rheumatoid arthritis 38, 40, 66–69
Rogers, Dr. Thomas 150
Ross, Dr. Ronald 90
Rutkow, Dr. Ira M. 109, 115, 118

salmonella 23, 35, 50, 88
sanitary reform movement 23
sanitation *xii*, 23–25, 28, 35–37
scarlet fever 120
scurvy 18, 28–29, 31, 40, 56–57, 114, 152
Semmelweis, Dr. Ignaz Philipp 19
septic arthritis 40, 58, 60–62, 85, 127–129
Shattuck, L. 23
shigella 35–36, 50, 88
Sickness and Mortality Reports 39, 48–49, 71, 80–81, 83, 112
smallpox 19, 112–113, 120, 136–138
Smart, Dr. Charles 45, 112
speculum 44
Stillé, Dr. Alfred 87, 93, 97, 99–100
streptococcal (strep) throat infection 40–43, 45, 47–49, 58, 61, 116, 120, 128
Sydenham, Dr. Thomas 50, 107
syphilis 40, 63–66, 87, 95, 106–108, 113, 116, 130

Index

tartar emetic 92, 102, 142–143
Tennessee 6th Infantry Regiment *xiii*, 112, 117
Tennessee 9th Infantry Regiment *xiii*, 112, 117
tonsillitis 31, 48–49, 122–124, 126
Transactions of the American Medical Association 110, 159
tuberculosis 38, 40, 45, 57–58, 74, 120, 135
turpeth mineral 103
typhoid fever 23, 31, 35, 38, 87–90, 93, 119

U. S. Sanitary Commission 103, 106, 130
   Inspectors 25, 39
   Reports 25, 48, 70, 93
University of Louisville Medical Department 18
University of Maryland School of Medicine 18
University of Pennsylvania School of Medicine *xiii*, 18–19, 60, 109–111, 134, 148, 153–154, 159
urethra *xii*, 40, 44, 50, 54, 63–64, 103, 119, 131

vaccination 19, 22, 112–113, 136–138
variola 120
variolation 112, 136
vital force (vitalism) 19, 155

Washington University Medical Department 18
Wassermann test 66, 106
Wöhler (Wohler), Friedrich 19
Wood, Dr. George Bacon 148–150, 153, 155, 158–159
Woodward, Dr. Joseph Janvier *xiii*, 25, 45, 54, 60, 90, 112, 115

yellow fever 119